Praise for
The Calm Birth Method

'Hypnobirthing expert and pregnancy coach Ashworth
has produced an excellent guide to the technique to
create a calm and positive birth experience. The book
explores the physiology and psychology of the mind and
body during pregnancy and birth to help women work
with the physiology of the birthing body rather than
against it, and is backed up with valuable breathing
exercises and visualizations alongside practical tools and
techniques to promote relaxation and mindfulness.'

YOGA MAGAZINE

'Having experienced anxiety in the past, I knew I wanted
to explore hypnobirthing to help me to feel calmer
about the whole experience. Reading The Calm Birth
Method has helped me to feel positive and even excited
about my upcoming birth. Highly recommended.'

CHLOE BROTHERIDGE, AUTHOR OF THE ANXIETY SOLUTION

'It is so good that it makes me miss labour. I have used
The Calm Birth School for all four of my births and I can
100 per cent recommend their hypnobirthing course. I am
kind of envious of those who are using this during their
pregnancy and labour now because it gave me such an
empowered and perfectly calm birth. Everyone deserves
that experience. If you want to feel empowered, in control
and powerful during and after labour then you need this.'

**SAMMI-JO, MULTI-AWARD WINNING DIGITAL
CREATOR, MOTHER FRESHLE**

'Take heed of Suzy Ashworth's advice. [She] shares tips for a positive labour, with mindful breathing techniques.'

BABY MAGAZINE

'Hypnobirthing expert Suzy Ashworth explores the physiology and psychology of the mind and body during pregnancy and birth in this new book. The author shares advice to promote relaxation and mindfulness, plus breathing techniques and visualizations to help with the birth process.'

YOUR HEALTHY LIVING MAGAZINE

The
Calm Birth
Method

The Calm Birth Method

NEW & UPDATED EDITION

Your Complete Guide to a
Positive Hypnobirthing Experience

SUZY ASHWORTH & LIZ STANFORD

HAY HOUSE
Carlsbad, California • New York City
London • Sydney • New Delhi

Published in the United Kingdom by:
Hay House UK Ltd, The Sixth Floor, Watson House,
54 Baker Street, London W1U 7BU
Tel: +44 (0)20 3927 7290; Fax: +44 (0)20 3927 7291
www.hayhouse.co.uk

Published in the United States of America by:
Hay House Inc., PO Box 5100, Carlsbad, CA 92018-5100
Tel: (1) 760 431 7695 or (800) 654 5126
Fax: (1) 760 431 6948 or (800) 650 5115
www.hayhouse.com

Published in Australia by:
Hay House Australia Ltd, 18/36 Ralph St, Alexandria NSW 2015
Tel: (61) 2 9669 4299; Fax: (61) 2 9669 4144
www.hayhouse.com.au

Published in India by:
Hay House Publishers India, Muskaan Complex, Plot No.3, B-2,
Vasant Kunj, New Delhi 110 070
Tel: (91) 11 4176 1620; Fax: (91) 11 4176 1630
www.hayhouse.co.in

A catalogue record for this book is available from the British Library.

Tradepaper ISBN: 978-1-4019-6666-9
E-book ISBN: 978-1-78817-721-4
Audiobook ISBN: 978-1-78817-717-7

Interior images: Suzy Ashworth

Printed in the United States of America

10 9 8 7 6 5 4 3 2 1

To the ones who started it –
Caesar, Coco and Aluna – I love you.

To Mike, Danni, Will and Jamie –
I do what I love because of you.

Contents

Acknowledgements

There are so many people to thank, acknowledge and consider when it comes to this book!

The biggest thank yous, of course, have to go to our families who have always put their belief in us to achieve our dreams! Our children were the reasons that both of us found hypnobirthing, which has ultimately led us here, to be able to help so many other women and birthing people to experience their births as positively as possible.

To all The Calm Birth School instructors past, present and future who help to spread the method and teachings across the world. The work you do is so, so important. You are changing the world, one birth at a time!

To Marie Mongan, where it all began, and to all the other creators of hypnobirthing programmes. Thank you for your continued passion for helping women, birthing people and families to experience calm and positive births.

To the amazing inspiring founders of Fivexmore who have literally made history with the impact of their grassroots organization. And to other organizations and people who are making huge leaps in creating safe spaces in birth preparation and maternity services for minorities and marginalized communities.

To all the contributors of our 'book bonuses', especially Anna Le Grange and Jade Gordon who are both doing fantastic work to help families navigate breastfeeding and parenting (respectively).

To all the birthers who have been through The Calm Birth School programme (either online or with an instructor) and have contributed their birth stories to this book. You motivate and inspire us and everyone who reads your words!

To all the birth workers out there... this can be a challenging but amazing field to work in. Thank you for continuing to do the work you do and prioritizing families as you do so.

And so there is only one other thank you to make here, and this is from Liz to Suzy. Thank you for trusting me to continue the work you started. I will be forever grateful and you will always be my fairy godmother.

Introduction:
No Vagina Whispering

So you've finally decided to bite the bullet, or maybe some kind soul decided to for you, and you want to know more about The Calm Birth Method (TCBM): the tools and techniques used in the world's first video-based hypnobirthing programme, The Calm Birth School (TCBS). Since its launch in December 2014, The Calm Birth Method family has helped nearly 10,000 birthing women and people across six different continents create calm and positive birth experiences, either via our video course or Liz's team of amazing instructors. TCBS instructors are passionate about working with pregnant women and people face to face (and online since the pandemic in 2020) and can be found across much of the world. You really are in the best company. But enough about us, let's cut to the chase and acknowledge the most important person in the room – that's you. Yes, you, who right now are growing another human being, even as you read these words. And that is by far the biggest deal in the world. You're bloody amazing!

Perhaps the whole 'growing a baby' thing is something that you've already got to grips with. If not, go google it. There are a million-and-one blogs and forums telling you exactly what size nut your baby is today. This book isn't about any of that, but rather the most amazing feat a pregnant woman or person's body ever goes through – giving birth. In the following chapters, you'll get the lowdown on all the different tips, tricks and techniques that have helped thousands of birthing women and people to have calm, empowering, positive and fear-free birth experiences.

Although this is primarily a book about giving birth, you'll also learn how to unleash your personal power from within, so that when the moment finally arrives for you to welcome your baby into the world, you'll feel calm, positive and ready for whatever twists and turns may be presented to you. The one thing we know for sure about birth is that it's a journey, and one where you can't know ahead of time exactly what's going to happen. You can, however, arm yourself with a mindset and a toolkit that can make giving birth one of the most incredible and enjoyable experiences of your life.

By the time you have finished reading this book, you'll understand exactly what you need to do to give yourself permission to go wherever you need to go, controlling what you can control and letting go of what you can't, as you eliminate the fear of birth. It's this inner confidence that will enable you to do what you need to do to bring your baby into the world positively, happily and powerfully.

Are we serious about birth being happy, positive and enjoyable? Absolutely. Are we those lentil-eating, hummus-knitting, crochet-knickers-wearing kind of women? Perhaps you'll be surprised to hear, we're not. Are we going to make you walk from room to room, wafting a joss stick while chanting in Sanskrit? Nope. (Liz is partial to a joss stick, but that's another story!) Will we be asking you to pay homage to the lotus flower or whisper to your vagina? No, no and no: there will be no vagina whispering! (Unless, of course, you want there to be.)

While we both secretly love all things a bit hippy and woo-woo, this book was originally written from Suzy's, let's-get-sh*t-done, pragmatic left brain and is updated with the same level of pragmatism, realism and enthusiasm. Between us, we have six children... six! Yes, that makes us raise our eyebrows too! And we are here to show you that no matter who you are, or what your perspective on birth, giving birth can be an experience you'll never forget – *for all the right reasons.*

While you might be feeling confident in your body's ability to do this job (and why the hell not? It is quite literally what your body is designed to do), it is also highly possible that you're peeing your pants at the thought of everything to do with the bit before you hold your baby in your arms for the first time.

If this is your first child, and you're anything like us, or many of The Calm Birth School clients, you might be in a bit of a head spin about having a baby growing inside you. That's OK. It's normal to get a bit freaked out as you comprehend that the collection of cells formulating within you right now – which started out smaller than a grain of rice – will one day become an actual human being. Both of us agree that it definitely fried our brains – even third time around!

Or perhaps the mere thought of squeezing a nine-pounder out of your nether regions brings tears to your eyes... so you aren't thinking about it. Maybe you're so busy being superhuman that the fact you're about to become a parent and give birth has barely registered on your inner Richter scale. You're just too goddamn busy right now to really give it any headspace. Or maybe you're the control freak who wants to know all the details. For you, the thought of your body doing things you can barely bring yourself to imagine makes you want to curl up under your duvet, so you're arming yourself with as much information as you can get. As we've said before, we at The Calm Birth School have been there and done this, and we work with women and people like you every day. We want you to know that it doesn't matter who you are or whether you're experienced or knowledgeable about birth: you really have got this.

By reading this book, you're acknowledging that at least a small part of you knows that birth doesn't have to be like the horror stories that are shown on TV, discussed with girlfriends/friends or overheard around the water cooler. You don't have to be that disempowered woman or person who feels scared, vulnerable and as though birth is happening *to* you. You don't have to go into labour unaware of all the things you don't know just because you haven't done this before.

The Calm Birth School's mission is to arm you with knowledge and empower you with confidence, so that you know from the core of your being that you were designed to do this. We are here to remind you that your innate ability to give birth – which has been genetically programmed into women and birthing people over hundreds of thousands of years – is right there at your fingertips.

Will this guarantee you an easy, straightforward birth during which your baby pops out reciting the alphabet backwards? (Hypno-babies are very advanced, you know.) Sadly, no. I wish I could guarantee such linguistic feats alongside a 'perfect' birth, but that isn't the case.

So what is the point of hypnobirthing then?

I'd like to invite you to think of your birth as the most important meeting of your life to date. What would you do before you knocked on the office door, ready to strut your stuff in front of your boss? You would prepare everything down to the nth degree. You would have every base covered so that whatever curveballs you might be faced with, you'd know you could handle it all. You'd feel calm, confident and ready to go.

You already know that as first meetings go, the date you have with your baby is going to be infinitely more impactful, meaningful and enjoyable than any meeting with a boss. My goal is for you to feel even more confident, prepared and knowledgeable than you would be if you were prepared to come face to face with the people who pay your salary.

Why is this so important? Well, contrary to popular opinion, we will declare unreservedly that giving birth should be one of the most empowering, life-affirming and joyful events you'll ever experience. When you learn to work with your body, as opposed to against it, you'll know how to embrace the sometimes weird, sometimes wonderful power and intensity that moves up, down, around and through your body. And when you allow yourself to go with that flow, knowing with every fibre of your being that you were born to do this, then yes, it really can feel amazing.

⋙ Natalie's birth story ⋘

To say I was worried about giving birth would be an understatement – I was petrified! If it hadn't been for my instructor Charlotte who was, literally, THE BEST, I don't think I would have felt as confident, amazing and ready to bring my baby into the world as I did.

Baby Ronnie decided to arrive a week early, and at the start of that week I'd been busy gutting my house! I was visiting a friend the day before I went into labour, but embarrassingly, I couldn't seem to get off her toilet. My friend googled this and apparently, it is sometimes a sign of labour starting. I started to get a little excited about the impending birth, but it was still early, and I thought, This isn't going to happen yet. Oh, how wrong I was!

I started to get seriously strong period-like cramps around 3 a.m. I decided to let my partner Aiden sleep a little longer, as I knew I would need him to be full of energy for what was about to come. What made the whole experience even more magical was, at this point, we still didn't know whether we were expecting a boy or a girl and I must admit, I was very excited about finding out.

As my labour progressed at home, I found it was comfortable at times to be sat on the toilet. As my waves got stronger, I also found that being on all fours on my sofa eased the pressure in my lower back. I messaged my midwife at 9 a.m. to let her know what was going on; then at 12:45 p.m. I messaged her to let her know my waters had released. Aiden and I danced around the living room when that happened!

I stayed at home for as long as possible, as I felt in control, relaxed and I was in a very good place emotionally. I could feel my body progressing and by 5:15 p.m. I felt it was time to go to hospital, as my waves were coming every two minutes.

Once at the birthing unit (with Aiden, who stayed by my side throughout), I was assessed, and it was music to my ears when I was informed I was 5cm dilated. I had the option of gas and air,[1] but I didn't really use it. I focused on my breathing techniques, and it helped that I had a midwife team that was out of this world.

My labour was exactly what I had hoped for. I was aware that things don't always go to plan, but throughout the whole experience I could feel my body adapting to the changes and every step was bringing me closer to the arrival of our baby. With the last few pushes, I actually felt below and touched my baby's hair, and I knew with one more push the head would be born. My body was made to do this. It was so natural – it felt like I had done it all before.

As my baby swam up to me in the birthing pool, it [felt as though everything was happening] in slow motion – I could see every small movement. I had my hands waiting to catch my baby – I was bursting with so much love. I was the happiest in the world, and I still am. The experience overall was incredible, and I cannot wait to do it again.

The calm birth experience is for you, of course, but it's also for your baby. When you release the resistance that can impede labour and birth, your baby's experience of entering the world becomes infinitely less jarring. A calm and positive end to your pregnancy and start to the newest chapter of your family's life enables you to focus on the most important job of all: getting to know this new little person who has just arrived. A positive, calm birth will also promote attachment and bonding with your baby, support you in being completely present at every precious moment of your newborn's life, and give you the emotional space that all new parents need to navigate the transition into parenthood.

The flipside of the above scenario is the negative, stressful or traumatic birth experience, which unfortunately we hear about all too often from second-time parents. Research shows that negative experiences during childbirth can lead to difficulties with bonding[2] and establishing breastfeeding (or chestfeeding).[3-4]

Hurt and anger are the feelings that many people describe when they look back at their birth experience. Often, they feel they were ignored or disempowered. This can also be coupled with feelings of isolation and guilt at not being able to express the disappointment of their experience, for fear of appearing ungrateful for the healthy baby they're holding in their arms. We hear stories of stress and angst from both parents as they try to make their way through the negative roller-coaster of emotions that a stressful birth experience can trigger.

These experiences can affect everyone, but are even more prevalent among minority races and communities. Although birth is considered to be very safe (please keep that in mind as you read the next few sentences), Black and Brown women and birthing people are much more likely than their white counterparts to experience a 'near miss'.[5] (We will delve into this in more detail later in the book.)

One study from 2014 shows that compared with white European women, Black African women are 83 per cent more likely and Black Caribbean women 80 per cent more likely to suffer a near miss. The reasons for these disparities and for others, have been shown to be linked to systemic racism. The number of LGBTQ+ parents having babies is currently unknown, but there is a steady increase year on year in the number of lesbian couples accessing fertility treatment and beginning or growing their families.[6] There are no figures available for the number of transgender people becoming pregnant or impregnating their partners.

There is also a lack of research into birth trauma when it comes to the LGBTQ+ community but there are Queer Birth workers and their allies working tirelessly to raise awareness of LGBTQ+ issues and the increasing need for more research and inclusion across the board. At the time of writing, no research into trans and non-binary parents' experiences has focused on birth trauma.[7]

We can't claim to resolve issues such as systemic racism and LGBTQ+ exclusion, nor can we wave away the trauma that anyone from any background, ethnicity or community has experienced. The message of this book is simple: birth shouldn't be a distressing experience – for anyone.

In this book, you'll learn:

- Simple but powerful tools and techniques to help you feel calm, confident and at ease during pregnancy and labour.

- How the mind–body connection can affect your ability to give birth optimally, and what you can do during your pregnancy to get it working for you, rather than against you.

- How to embrace your pregnant self and why it is important for your birth.

- How you can get your care providers working with you for your specific needs, so that you feel like you're the one running the show during your pregnancy and birth, no matter where and how you give birth.

- Some great ways to get your birth partner involved in your pregnancy, so they feel equipped to support you and be your advocate on the day.

I can't emphasize enough how important your birth partner will be during this process, so if you know it's going to be an uphill challenge getting them to read this book with you, I highly recommend The Calm Birth School video course or going even deeper and working with one of our lovely TCBS instructors. The online course comes with a private students' Facebook group, which means, if you need it, you get personalized support from Liz and the other students in there.

Working with an instructor, either in a group or one-to-one format, online or in person, means that you get a tailored experience and can expect a top-class service. Depending on your circumstances, you may want to choose an instructor who has undergone additional training in topics such as Anti-racism, LGBTQ+ Competency or Birth Trauma Competency. These are indicated by 'buttons' located on our instructors' directory, their own websites or social media platforms. Check out all the details for the video programme at www.thecalmbirthschool.com/course and find a TCBS instructor local to you, or www.thecalmbirthschool.com/instructor-directory/ to find one you can work with online.

Whether you read the following chapters alongside either of the above options or as a standalone, you'll finish this book feeling uber-prepared for the most important day of your life.

Ready to get started?

Let's do this!

Suzy and Liz xo

How to Use This Book

Maybe you have a huge pile of pregnancy and birth books on your bedside table, or perhaps this is the only book you intend to read before your baby arrives. (There are a million other things you could be doing, right? After all, reading lots of pregnancy and birth books makes everything a bit *too* real, doesn't it?) Either way, this is the most important book you'll read about creating a positive birth experience.

Within the following chapters and the amazing The Calm Birth School Community Group on Facebook, you'll not only find the tools you need for an amazing birth, but also a philosophy to take into your life. You'll gain a better understanding of what you can control and what you can't, develop an enhanced appreciation of the difference between flow and resistance, and understand what you need to do to adjust your environment to suit you and your baby. Starting today, and while reading this book, you'll gain a newfound inner confidence and experience your unique ability to tune in to the changes within your body as it grows with your baby. This will make it even easier to understand exactly what you and your family will require to create the best possible foundation for the most positive birth experience that you deserve and desire.

To get the most out of this book, it is best to read each section, practise the exercises and do homework as you go along. While it might be tempting to skim-read, solely looking for the techniques for labour, The Calm Birth Method (TCBM) takes a holistic approach to learning, so if you only look for the bits about 'how to breathe', for example, you won't do yourself or your birth justice. I wish it could be as easy as saying 'read and breathe and you'll be fine', but it doesn't work like that. I know that when you practise these techniques they will work, and not just because we have used them during our own births, but because thousands of other people have successfully used this exact same process, too.

The line in the sand is clear when it comes to understanding those birthing women and people who benefit most from these tools. The secret is, it's not really a secret. The joyful stories come from those who put time into completing the homework and tuning in to the belief that they can create a positive birth experience, regardless of whether their baby decides to follow their birth preferences to the letter or has other ideas.

The clients who asked questions, invested in The Calm Birth School course (online or with an instructor), bought books, did their research and, in some cases, got extra support when they needed it, focused on and strengthened their ability to create a positive birth experience.

Please note that at no point will I say that 'positive' equals 'perfect'. Your birth doesn't have to be quick, straightforward or textbook for you to have an amazing experience. As you'll see from the array of birth stories in this book – which include caesarean births, home births, hospital births, long births and very quick births – and everything in between – each person's experience is different. And it all starts with how you think and speak about giving birth to your baby.

The language of birth and the importance of inclusivity

The language you use and hear about birth is especially important because it can make a real difference to whether you feel calm or anxious about the prospect of giving birth. The reason for this is that words have the power to evoke huge emotional responses. A kind word can make the stress of a horrible day fade in seconds, while another person might get your blood boiling by stating something that wouldn't register with anyone else. For example, someone might say to a pregnant parent-to-be, 'So are you going back to work once you've had the baby, or are you just going to be a stay-at-home mum?'

The word 'just' is often enough to trigger stress in many pregnant women and people, as it suggests that being a full-time parent is less worthy or important than going back to paid employment. To take this one step further, if someone doesn't identify as a woman (perhaps they are a trans-man or a non-binary individual) then the word 'mum' could also be triggering here. At The Calm Birth School, we believe that our methods and message should be accessible to all who might need to prepare to birth a baby. This is why you'll have already read words like 'birthing people' and 'pregnant people' in addition to the word 'woman'. This isn't the act of cancelling out one word for another. It is merely using terms to include everyone who might be accessing this book, or using the correct terms for an individual when face to face with them. The reason is simple – words create imagery in the mind, which, in turn, triggers emotions. In fact, every thought we have creates a chemical and physical response in the body, and we'll be exploring this in more detail in a later chapter.

From this point onwards, I would like you to minimize your exposure to some of the more negative words or phrases about giving birth (and explore which words impact you the most) by replacing them with the more positive Calm Birth School terms, shown below:

Instead of saying...	Say...
Contraction	Wave or surge
Broken (as in waters)	Released
Pain	Discomfort, sensations or pressure
Birth canal	Birth path
Pushing	Bearing down
Complications	Special circumstances
C-section	Caesarean birth or abdominal birth
Natural birth	Vaginal birth

For now, just notice how it feels to say or hear the word(s) in the left-hand column compared to the one(s) on the right.

Preparing for birth

Feeling calm about the prospect of giving birth is one of the key tools of The Calm Birth School, and you'll be learning many practices in this book to help you achieve it, but one of the other key tools is being prepared.

So, how are you going to prepare for your birth? If you want the kind of birth that is available for you, you'll make a commitment now to do your homework and participate in the online group.

As you go through the book, highlight all the parts that stand out as important to you and those that will be useful for your partner to read. Even though you're the one having the baby, it's really important that your birth partner gets involved too, as they will play a vital role in ensuring that everything is set up as you need it to be. Your partner also needs to have a clear understanding of TCBS techniques – what to use and when, and how to encourage and support you – without the worry of you morphing into an angry fireball. We've all heard those stories about birthing women and people in labour who threaten physical violence to anyone within arm's reach. Your partner's preparation is vitally important and will enable them to be the best support for you, alongside providing them with their own set of tools to fall back on. Witnessing this miraculous event is no small matter and when emotions are running high, 'your' hypnobirthing tools will be as invaluable to your partner as they are to you.

If you're experiencing a low-risk pregnancy, hypnobirthing will help you to create a firm foundation for enjoying a vaginal birth with no intervention, although, of course, this isn't guaranteed. This is why reading the entire book is important: I want you to be at ease with the idea that you can navigate any situation you're presented with in a way that leaves you feeling positive, confident and in control of your birth, rather than the birth being 'something that happens to you'.

> ## — Tip —
>
> Listening to The Calm Birth School audio downloads daily will turbocharge your learning and confidence. You can purchase these via www.thecalmbirthschool.com/shop/ or listen to the Calm Birth Hypnobirthing Meditation via the *Empower You: Unlimited Audio* mobile app.
>
> In addition, you can visit www.thecalmbirthschool.com/the-calm-birth-school-book-bonuses/ to download your free 'practice schedule'.

Once you're into the final four weeks of your pregnancy, it's a good idea to read the book again, step up your breathing and visualization practices, and you'll be good to go.

So as we prepare to dive in, remember: positive does not have to mean perfect.

❧ Zoe's birth story ❧

I went into spontaneous labour Saturday daytime (after my 'bloody show', which started Friday). During the early stages, we passed the time with a long walk (crazy I know, but I wanted to go!), followed by a bath, an early dinner and a party (so my three-year-old named it). We had fairy lights up, we danced and continued to be jolly. Around 8:30 p.m., I decided it was time to ring my mum to collect my daughter and to put my TENS machine on. As Alex was attaching the TENS machine, my waters went! We continued to labour at home, listening to the hypnobirthing audio downloads until my surges were about three minutes apart. We decided it was time to make our way to hospital at that point. My surges continued in the car, but when we reached the hospital, they slowed right down.

The midwife, before examining me, said, 'I'm not sure you're in active labour as you haven't had a surge since you arrived,' (about fifteen minutes). I was not impressed, but she then examined me and said I was a good 7cm dilated – Ha! She was surprised, as I was so calm, and said I could use the birth pool when it was ready – Brilliant!

I continued to labour in the room, listening to Bob Marley on a speaker out loud. I combined this with the hypnobirthing audio downloads playing in my earphones.

The water was amazing! I was so, so calm. The midwife commented a few times that I didn't look [as though I was] in labour... I guess I was too chilled (if that's possible)! Labour was slow, but very calm. At around 5 a.m. they asked me to get out of the pool for an examination, as not much was happening. I was over 9cm dilated, but not quite 10. I had a pocket of forewaters in front of the baby's head. The midwife felt this [was] maybe slowing things down, so we decided to release the pocket. This certainly helped, but as soon as I entered the pool, labour slowed again. I decided to stand up to encourage surges... this worked! I got out of the pool and started having the urge to push. This was a strange sensation – from nothing to this! I stayed out of the pool until the surges were building up to a point where they looked like they wouldn't stop again.

I re-entered the pool, and had the urge to push again straight away. It took about ten to twelve pushes... with each one I was focused on relaxing my jaw and breathing. Entering the world slowly was probably the best thing [for my baby, and for me]. It was calm and I was able to push out a very large baby with only a very small tear. He weighed 10lb (with a 39cm head circumference). He had a very calm entry to the world, so thank you.

We definitely had the birth we wanted.

CHAPTER 1

What Is Hypnobirthing?

When addressing the question of what hypnobirthing is, it's probably best to start with what hypnobirthing isn't. Hypnobirthing isn't hocus-pocus. As hypnotherapists we laugh in the face of the idea of 'mind control'... seriously, that is *not* hypnobirthing. The good news is that you won't find yourself barking uncontrollably every time you see a full moon or dry-humping your birth partner in a room full of strangers for comic entertainment. Hypnobirthing has nothing to do with witchcraft (although we aren't opposed to being a little witchy!) and everything to do with science.

So if it's not mind control or witchcraft, what is it? Quite simply, hypnobirthing enables you to feel calm and connected to your baby during your pregnancy, and can provide you with invaluable tools and techniques that will allow you to stay relaxed during your birth. By the time you have completed this book – if you practise what we're going to teach you – you'll be the equivalent of a Jedi Master at instant relaxation whatever the situation, using your breath to feel calm and at ease, as well as utilizing visualization to help increase your focus.

Alongside the tangible hypnobirthing tools are the equally important, yet more intangible elements, which also impact your birthing journey. These present themselves in different ways for different people, but the common thread that underpins the change many Calm Birth School students outline is a newfound confidence, self-belief in the birthing process, faith in your body and not being afraid to share those beliefs with others. The Calm Birth School's approach to hypnobirthing aims to create the most positive birth experience for you, your baby and everyone involved in your birth.

ஐ **Vanessa's birth story** ஐ

One day past my 'guess' date, I had woken a few times during the night with backache. I thought nothing of this, putting it down to the usual pregnancy aches and pains!

When I woke at 6:30 a.m. I felt waves of period-like pains coming and going. They were quite frequent (about one or two every 10 minutes), so I presumed it was most likely Braxton Hicks.

I had some breakfast and decided to go back to bed for a lie-down. While upstairs at about 8 a.m., I decided to try and change position during one of these pains, to see if it would go away. This would have reassured me that it was Braxton Hicks. I got on my hands and knees in bed, ready to move. All of a sudden I felt a pop! A huge gush of waters went all over our bed!

I called my husband up from downstairs and told him things had definitely started. I then went to the bathroom and called my midwife while sat on the toilet.

My husband told me at this point that my waters had a black/green tinge to them. I told the midwife this and she said we would have to go into triage. She explained that if it cleared, we could still come home and have our home birth.

In my head, though, I kind of knew that if we went into hospital, we wouldn't be coming back out again. I think I made my peace then and there that I would likely not get the home birth I had planned. It had been touch and go so many times during the COVID-19 pandemic. I had been so happy when home births had started up once more, but I knew this was always a chance. So we moved onto Plan B.

My husband was on and off the phone to Lucy, our doula, who gave him amazing support and reassurance. I was sick a couple of times and the surges were increasing in intensity. Lucy helped him to help me through this.

Time started to pass very quickly. I realized afterwards that it was over two hours before I got in the car to go to the hospital. I had a TENS machine on. We breathed through each surge. I pictured my positive affirmations in my head:

'I can do anything for one minute.'

'Every surge brings my baby closer to me.'

'I feel safe, I feel calm. My body and baby know what to do.'

When we got to the hospital, my husband wasn't allowed into triage. I was in there for an hour and my surges ramped up a lot during that time. My husband again was able to speak with Lucy while he waited. This helped him stay calm while separated from me.

I asked to use the pool and was told that due to the meconium in my waters, I could not go to the

Midwife-Led Unit (MLU). Instead, I would need to stay on the labour ward.

I asked for gas and air. I was asked to consent to a vaginal examination (VE) to see if I was in established labour. If so, they could move me to the labour ward where gas and air was available. I had stated in my birth plan I did not want any VEs. However, I was confident I was in established labour. I wanted to move out of triage and have my husband back with me. I also wanted to get some gas and air for the intensity of the surges. Using my BRAIN (Benefit / Risk analysis) I decided to consent.

I was told I was 4cm and fully effaced. Plus, my surges were coming three in 10 minutes. I was moved quickly to the labour ward and my husband was allowed in. This was around 11 a.m.

Things continued to ramp up quickly. Really focusing on my breathing helped. My affirmations were helping a lot as the surges got to four or five every 10 minutes and strong in intensity. I felt like I should get off my back and onto my hands and knees and I also felt like I should go to the toilet. I could feel myself giving little pushes with each surge but felt that something was blocking baby's head from moving downwards.

By this stage, every time I tried to move another surge would take over. Things get a bit hazy time-wise here, but I remember hearing the doctor talking about putting in a canula and wanting to put a clip on my baby's head to monitor her. I declined all of this (and my husband was amazing at holding the pushy doctor off!).

As a result, I was asked to consent to another VE. I decided to agree to this because my intuition was telling me that everything was fine. My intuition told me we'd be meeting our baby soon and I felt it would stop the pressure for these interventions. I told them I didn't want to know what the result was, even though again I felt sure I had to be pretty far along. However, I heard the doctor come back into the room shortly after and say to a midwife that I was 9cm. This actually really helped me find the focus I needed for the last hour or so.

The midwife told me that they thought my full bladder was preventing baby's head from coming down. This made sense to me, from what I was feeling myself. Again, I used my BRAIN to decide to consent to an in/out catheter to drain my bladder. I knew I couldn't make it to the toilet myself and it would help my baby to descend.

Sure enough, as soon as they did this, my surges kicked into overdrive. I could feel her head moving rapidly downwards. I shifted onto my side and my husband helped prop my leg up. This was a great position for giving my pelvis more space while still allowing me to lie down.

Our daughter Isla was born shortly afterwards at 3:05 p.m. weighing 8lb 1½oz. She was perfect in every way. We had 10 minutes of delayed cord clamping, immediate skin-to-skin and I breastfed her while still in the labour ward. My husband had skin-to-skin with her while I had a few stitches for a very minor tear.

We tried for a physiological third stage. After waiting 40 minutes, I was fed up and wanted to get out of there. I agreed to a managed third stage and had the injection, birthing a HUGE placenta shortly afterwards!

We thought my husband would have to go straight home after. I had been told I would need to stay in for 12 hours of observations for baby because of the meconium in the waters. Amazingly, the midwives found us a room on the MLU and my husband was allowed to stay the entire time with us. We stayed there overnight all together and got home the next day at 3 p.m.

Our birth was very different to what we had planned, but it was a really positive experience. We had the confidence from the hypnobirthing course we did. We declined those interventions we felt were unnecessary and adapted our birth preferences according to the situation we found ourselves in, using our BRAIN to make decisions.

Our baby is happy, healthy and amazingly calm. I put this down to staying calm and relaxed throughout my pregnancy.

How do you create your own calm birth?

It's rare that we see others giving birth in Western society today. Labour tends to be a secretive event that takes place hidden away in a hospital room or in your own home. This huge shift towards privacy has really only come about in the last 50 years or so, but it has made an unimaginably massive difference in the way we view and experience birth. It is likely that you'll never have seen someone in labour until you're in labour yourself!

This has left us in an interesting place. For many, the only insight we get into one of the most significant rites of passage will come from the TV or movies, where it's often sensationalized, dramatized and presented as a torturous experience: a birthing woman or person lies on their back, face screwed up in agony, screaming, pushing and writhing in pain until a baby comes out. This has skewed our perception of what labour is like. We go into birth fearing the worst because, let's be honest, most of the time, what we have seen in the media looks bloody horrendous. Our sanitized culture has also invited us to be squeamish and recoil from anything involving bodily fluids.

On the rare occasion that we remember that we're actually mammals, we might look at how other warm-blooded animals give birth, in a documentary, for example. It's easy to see an animal's four legs compared to our two and to assume that birth is going to be easier, quicker and less painful for animals because 'we humans are just built differently'.

The problem with this assumption is that it's just plain wrong. Our physical design is not the issue. If that was the case, how do you explain the thousands of birthing women and people who give birth every year using hypnobirthing techniques – often without any pain relief – who recall their births as easy, comfortable and joyful? You may be tempted to write off those experiences by saying they have higher pain thresholds, bigger pelvises, gave birth to smaller babies or any other excuse – I mean, story – which springs to mind. These are, however, not the real reasons why some birth experiences are so empowering. There is more at work here.

While the wide-scale medicalization of birth means we are fortunate to be able to tap into world-class medical expertise in the West, it also means more opt to birth in hospitals rather than at home. Where once birth was witnessed many times as mothers, sisters and friends gave birth, the experience was thought of as normal and natural, nowadays birth is often perceived as a mysterious, scary and necessary evil, one we have to endure to get to the 'good bit' at the end. This has left us feeling less confident about our ability to give birth – a job we were made for – without medical intervention and assistance.

There is a simple reason why someone who doesn't do the type of preparation you're about to undertake will be unlikely to give birth in the same way as any other birthing mammal on the planet – comfortably, calmly and without fear. This reason has nothing to do with design features. In fact, for low-risk, straightforward pregnancies, the pleasant delivery of a newborn has everything to do with what's going on in your mind as you prepare for and give birth. The real issue is in the mind, not the body. Now that we know this, we can address it.

The evolution of birth

When we look at evolution, physiology and the fact that birthing women and people have ensured the survival of the human race over the last 200,000 years, it's fair to say we have done a pretty good job, right? Our ancestors somehow instinctively knew how to give birth. It would have been perceived as an everyday life event, which demystified it and stopped it from being scary. This genetic wisdom has been imprinted in your DNA and we see it as The Calm Birth School's job to provide you with the tools and techniques you need to access that information. This is knowledge that you have always had at your fingertips, but which has been drowned out by the cultural noise we've lived with in Western society in recent decades. Luckily, there's no rocket science involved in getting tuned in, but we do need to get a bit scientific.

Biology and neuroscience

Neither of us are scientists, but the fundamentals of hypnobirthing and how it works are based on the biology of the body and the science of the brain, otherwise known as neuroscience.

For the vast majority of birthing women and people, the instinctive response to the onset of labour is physical and emotional stress. This stress response is triggered in the limbic system, which sits in the oldest part of the brain, formed around 200,000–250,000 years ago.

When we look back to those times, the most important aspects of human life were reproduction and survival (some argue that they still are). Language did not play a role in life; everything was based on the messages we received via our five senses of sight, touch, sound, taste and scent. These cues triggered chemical and physiological changes within the body, determining how we felt and what we needed to do, whether that meant running for our lives, fighting to the death, or freezing and pretending we were dead to protect ourselves.

The part of the brain responsible for logical, rational thinking and critical analysis, the neocortex, didn't even exist at this point. Life centred on the instinctive responses needed for survival, in order to protect ourselves from the dangers and threats of the outside world. But this ancient hardwiring is still present in us now. The limbic system continues to protect us from danger in exactly the same way today as it did hundreds of thousands of years ago. When we perceive a danger cue (whether it's real or imaginary) the limbic system, which is designed to keep us safe, wins in the fight between instinct and thinking about the best course of action logically. In short, it overrides the neocortex and tips us into fight–flight–freeze mode.

When we bring this back to the context of birth, although most of us in the West aren't facing life-or-death scenarios, the fear that arises when giving birth inevitably triggers the fight–flight–freeze response. In turn, this sets off a physiological reaction, stress hormones adrenaline and cortisol flood the body (don't worry, we'll go into the role they play within birth later in the book), and the automatic emotional chain of events this sets off is what can prevent us from birthing optimally in the way we were designed to do.

Part of TCBM approach to hypnobirthing is ensuring that you understand how to minimize the fight–flight–freeze response by working with the biology of your body, instead of against it. In addition, this approach will help you to start thinking and feeling differently about the expectations you have around birth. This will support you before, during and after the actual act of giving birth.

The neuroscience bit

I'm guessing you've heard about a technique called 'visualization'. This is another one of those words that people sometimes think is a bit 'out there' or New Age. However, it is to become a vital tool in your hypnobirthing journey and you'll find masses of information, evidence and case studies on it if you look at psychology and the science of sport.

Before Tiger Woods became known as 'the adulterer', he was widely acclaimed as the greatest golfer the world had ever seen – and he is an avid visualizer. You might also have heard of Jim Carrey. Idris Elba? What about Will Smith? David Beckham? Eddie Izzard? Oprah? Come on now, you must have heard of Oprah! Seriously though, all these multimillion-dollar high achievers have spoken widely on the power of visualization. So what has this got to do with how you can give birth calmly, comfortably and more positively? It's all about your wiring.

Whether you see something in real life or simply imagine it, the combination of what you perceive and how you feel about what you perceive creates what is known as a 'neural pathway' in your brain. This pathway helps you determine how you're going to respond to stimuli that come your way. Think of it as a blueprint that your brain calls upon when you're faced with a situation where you feel threatened.

When it comes to birth, whether you have consciously thought about your forthcoming experience or not, you'll have seen many negative images and depictions of what birth is going to be like. Even before pregnancy, you may have already created a less-than-wonderful birthing blueprint and, whether it is based on fact or fiction, this can draw your body into fight–flight–freeze mode because it triggers the suggestion that there is danger; a need for fear or concern about your ability to birth effectively and efficiently. This gets overridden if you have witnessed or been a part of a positive birth experience, when a new blueprint can be formed through exposure to new stimuli.

David Beckham, Tiger Woods, Andy Murray, Katie Ledecky and many other high achievers and performers use visualization to create the ideal blueprint of their role within the game or in the tournament before it has actually happened. They teach themselves how to kick or hit the ball at the perfect trajectory in their minds, many, many times. Then, when the time comes to step out onto the pitch, golf course, court or swimming pool, their brains instinctively know where to go because their present situation feels so familiar. This isn't a new situation to them; they have already visited the scene many times through visualization. And because they are familiar with it, they don't have to deal with the same levels of adrenaline and cortisol, which come from being plonked into an unfamiliar scenario. The fight–flight–freeze response doesn't kick in, which in turn allows them to perform at the peak of their potential.

This stuff works just as effectively in a labour room, but there is more on how to use this technique in the next chapter.

Let's look at what else you're going to learn and take action on:

- How to manage the instinctive fight–flight–freeze response.

- How to minimize your physiological and emotional responses to stress.

- How to promote oxytocin and endorphin production (your feel-good hormones) to aid the process of birth.

- How to create the optimal environment for giving birth.

- How to ensure your birth partner can work confidently with you and your care providers.

The key element that ties everything together is learning how to relax. Sounds good, right? It is. Let's keep going; there's a lot to cover!

CHAPTER 2

An Introduction to Relaxation

M indfulness and meditation are buzzwords nowadays, and have entered the mainstream in a major way. In 2019, the UK government invested funds to study the benefits of mindfulness in children's classrooms.[8] This was after almost a decade of other work to bring mindfulness into schools across the UK (such as pledging £1 million per year to training teachers to teach mindfulness to children) while global organizations such as Apple, Google, Nike and even the UK Home Office have embraced mindfulness training for their employees. The constant drip feed of information on social media about mindfulness means that most of us know that learning to switch off and still the mind will benefit us, but we just can't bring ourselves to do it.

The fear of missing out on what's going on in cyberspace often robs us of invaluable time that we need to be by ourselves.[9] Believe it or not, you need to come at the top of the priority list during pregnancy, followed by your loved ones, family and friends, with the social media world at the very bottom of the list.

Taking time out for you

The first thing we invite – no, challenge – you to do during your pregnancy is to start deliberately taking time for you. In an ideal world, you'll enjoy some quiet time for 30 minutes, just focusing on your breath at least once a day. That means no television, no phone, no laptop, not even a book: just time and space where you give yourself permission to let your mind have a break from thinking, analysing, planning and doing. If things pop into your mind during this time, acknowledge them, tell them you'll address them later, and bring your attention back to your breath.

Some of you will read that and think, 'Hell no! That sounds hideous!' Others will think, 'Yes, that sounds great, but back in the real world...'. I get it. You're busy. However, you're also pregnant. You're growing new life inside you.

— Tip —

If 30 minutes' downtime feels overwhelming or unrealistic right now, start with less – say 15 minutes – and use the following ideas to help get you started:

~ Spend 15 minutes doing nothing before you get out of bed, focusing only on your breath using one of the breathing techniques you're about to learn.

~ Break the rest of your alone time down into five-minute chunks by getting unplugged three times throughout the day and focusing on nothing but regulating your breathing.

~ If you find it hard to get time alone owing to the demands of work or small children, or both, pick a quiet moment and lock yourself in the bathroom for five minutes, where you're less likely to be disturbed.

There are lots of reasons why having some downtime to yourself is good for you and your baby, so don't resist it. You're reading this book to give yourself the best possible foundation for creating a positive birth experience for you and your little bundle of fun, and the preparation starts here, oddly, with choosing to do nothing.

It's a pretty good gig and if I haven't hammered home the message enough, here follow all the reasons why:

1. Lower stress levels – this is a BIG deal

A lot of people work or live with more than their fair share of stress. When you take the time to switch off, it actively lowers the amount of the stress hormone, cortisol, in your blood. You'll appreciate this in ways you might not even notice, but trust me, low cortisol levels are a good thing. Your baby agrees, too.

2. More effective thinking

When we're stressed or angry, we become stupid. I'm being blunt but fair here. We find it difficult to think rationally or creatively when we're in a stressed-out state and are essentially useless at problem-solving. That's why TCBS breathing technique is especially useful when you're in a stressful situation at work (you'll learn how to use this technique a little later in this chapter). Ideally, you would excuse yourself from the problem, go to the lavatory and do a bit of TCBS breathing, to create the mental space to come up with a solution. Even if you can't excuse yourself, the simple act of remaining silent and focusing on your breath will help you disengage from the frustration and be more proactive rather than reactive.

3. Pain control

There is increasing evidence to suggest that the more we can disengage from our surroundings, such as when we go into a meditative state of mind, our pain receptors become less sensitive.[10]

4. Induces emotional calm

Not only can you handle stressful situations more easily, but also you don't get riled as often either. Stressful situations roll off you like water off a duck's back, which is good for you, good for your family and amazing for your baby.

The feedback I have received from clients is that the TCBS breathing techniques aren't just indispensable during birth but also tools that you can draw on after your baby arrives. Being able to stay calm when you feel completely responsible for this new little life, while simultaneously being completely out of your comfort zone, is an invaluable life skill. Start putting yourself first today and embracing the downtime that is oh so good for you.

··

The Calm Birth School breathing technique

··

The reason TCBS breathing technique is so effective is that your out-breath is nearly twice as long as your in-breath, and this triggers your body's natural calming reflex. During labour this breathing technique will help you maintain a deep state of calm and you can use it in between surges to help you remain calm and focused. You'll also use it as you feel a surge (contraction) coming in and once it has subsided.

Ideally, the breath is taken in and out through the nose as opposed to the mouth as this gives you more control over the flow of air. However, please don't stress if you have a cold when you're birthing. Just breathe through your mouth – it will all be OK.

How to do it

1. Breathe in deeply to the count of four through your nose.

2. As you breathe in, imagine filling your lungs right to the bottom.

3. As you breathe out, imagine sending the breath down, so it moves around your baby, down your legs and into the tips of your toes, and then into the floor, before breathing out to the count of seven.

When you're learning to use this technique, you might find it helpful to place your hands on your waist, so that you can feel the rise and fall of your abdomen as you breathe deeply. It really is as simple as that.

If you find it difficult to increase your out-breath for a count of seven, simply reduce your exhalation to a number that feels comfortable, or increase the pace. As you start to feel more relaxed, you can either up your count or increase your pace. The most important thing is not to worry if it doesn't all come together immediately. The act of bringing conscious awareness to your breathing during your pregnancy will help you once you go into labour.

When to do it

Ensure you do at least one set of TCBS breathing in the morning for five minutes, five minutes at lunchtime and five minutes again in the evening. In addition, use this technique whenever you feel stressed, whether it is at work, with your partner, getting on or off public transport – wherever and whenever. The more you practise TCBS breathing technique, the quicker it will become your automatic response to stress.

That last point is particularly important if you labour quickly, as this breathing technique will get you into the birthing zone quickly and easily.

If you tend to take life in your stride with very little stress, this doesn't make you exempt from practising this breathing technique. It's just as important that you carve out some practice time for your TCBS breathing, too.

As you get better and better at using TCBS breathing technique, you'll notice how the skill of being able to relax on demand – and eventually very, very deeply – becomes both instinctive and invaluable to you. And by the time you reach your labour day, you'll be able to relax and enjoy (yes – enjoy!) the process, as your ability to release stress and tension from your body in everyday life will help you to learn to trust that your body will be able to do this for you during your labour when you need it to the most.

....

Hypnosis/trance

In many cases, people feel weird about hypnosis (which is often referred to as trance, and I will use the two terms interchangeably). The sense of weirdness often comes from what they have seen on stage and TV shows. While this type of hypnosis often makes for great entertainment, it is completely misleading and incredibly frustrating for anyone who uses hypnosis in a therapeutic setting, because what we see on TV or on stage is an illusion: the illusion of mind control.

Let me explain what I mean. The first thing anyone working in hypnotherapy is taught is that all hypnosis is self-hypnosis. This means that you can't make anyone do anything that doesn't sit comfortably with them. When we watch a stage hypnotist, what we're seeing is an audience made up of two kinds of people: those who are there to be entertained and those who are there to be the entertainment. We'll see a large group of people invited up onto the stage and they'll be directed to participate in 'entertaining' things that usually involve them looking a bit silly. As the show goes on, the suggestions that the stage hypnotist uses will become increasingly outrageous.

Every single person up there will have their own internal barometer that tells them when enough is enough. As each reaches that point, you'll notice them choosing not to participate on the stage, and at that point the hypnotist will tap them on the shoulder and ask them to sit down. Finally, you're left with the 'star' of the show – the person who feels the least inhibited in that environment, doing things that under normal circumstances they wouldn't want their grandmother to watch. At no point can anyone be forced to do anything they do not want to do, and the only reason that they are clucking like a chicken or barking like a dog on demand is because they want to.

I hope that sets the record straight once and for all: hypnosis has nothing to do with mind control!

So if hypnosis isn't mind control, what is it?

Hypnosis is a natural state of consciousness we drift in and out of whenever we have a narrowed focus of attention or are deeply relaxed in passive or active activity. It's a state that we all drift in and out of naturally at least 10–12 times every single day. The times you'll be most familiar with are when you're just drifting off to sleep or when you're just waking up.

Other examples of natural states of trance include:

- daydreaming
- running
- dancing
- sex
- drawing, colouring or any other creative pursuit, e.g. writing, pottery, sewing, etc.
- driving a familiar route, e.g. to work or to the local shops
- watching a great movie
- listening to someone tell a story.

We enter trance whenever we experience a narrowed focus of attention, becoming deeply absorbed in an activity that we are very familiar with or are extremely relaxed doing; the logical part of our mind becomes more easily sidetracked. Whenever the brain isn't required to critically analyse everything we are doing, a gap in our thinking is created, and this leaves us more open to suggestion. This state of suggestibility can't occur when we are learning a new skill or taking part in an activity that requires us to be alert and aware.

This is really important to remember if you find yourself listening intently to someone else's birth story, particularly if it is about a terrible experience. The more involved and engaged you become with the story, the more open to suggestion you become. In this type of scenario your brain stops critically acknowledging that the story you're hearing is only the specific storyteller's experience, and without realizing it you start to file the information under the 'What is True About Birth' file in your brain's hard drive. As the suggestion that birth is an awful and scary experience gets implanted in your brain through listening to this tale, it becomes your point of reference when you think about birth and, most importantly, when you go into labour.

Therefore, it is imperative that you consciously avoid listening to negative birth stories at any opportunity – even if that means removing yourself from the conversation. However, the upside of this is pretty great, as the fact that you're more open to suggestion and to storing information in your brain's database when you feel calm, relaxed or focused is exactly what we capitalize on when it comes to your hypnobirthing journey. This is the exact reason why hypnosis is so great for helping you to retrain your mind about how to think and feel about birth. It can be used just as effectively to reinforce positive suggestions, feelings and associations you have about your upcoming labour and birth.

So let's bust some hypnosis myths:

- **You can get 'stuck' in hypnosis:** You can't get stuck in hypnosis in the same way that it's impossible to get stuck in sleep!

- **Hypnosis is harmful:** The only time hypnosis can be harmful is when a person is in a natural state of trance, listening uncritically to someone else's suggestions about an event, such as in the example given above, when you find yourself listening to someone else's negative birth story without acknowledging that the experience being recounted does not have to have any bearing on the way that you give birth.

- **Hypnosis is mind control:** Well, we've already busted that one! Remember: all hypnosis is self-hypnosis.

The brain

While we're not going to dive deep into the truly fascinating world of neuroscience, understanding the basics of how your brain works will help you get clear on why going into a state of trance, self-hypnosis or meditation by yourself is so great for birth.

I'd like you to imagine the brain being like an iceberg. The tip of the iceberg is where all of our logical, rational thinking takes place, but the subconscious, which is effectively all the stuff going on beneath the surface, is where most of the action is.

The subconscious mind runs our autonomic nervous system and is responsible for the beating of our heart, the blinking of our eyes and anything we do without consciously thinking about it. It is also the home of our emotions, our imagination and where our gut feeling, intuition or 'sixth sense' originates.

The driving force behind everything our subconscious does is ultimately designed to keep us safe. The way it does this is by keeping records or memories – both visually and emotionally – of everything we have ever seen or been a part of, and categorizing them crudely as either 'safe' or 'unsafe'. If an event takes place for which we don't have a frame of reference (in other words, a brand-new experience), the subconscious will look for the most similar thing we have experienced and then trigger a set of physical and emotional responses in line with that reference point.

An example of this might be someone witnessing another person getting hit by a car. If they haven't been able to process the incident logically, the memory of seeing the accident will trigger a chain of physiological and emotional responses, which might result in the subconscious telling the person instinctively, 'It's no longer safe to cross the road.'

This is what happens so frequently when it comes to birth. Unless you have experienced a difficult birth, the majority of people will have only witnessed challenging births on TV or heard other people's stories. Birth stories, and more specifically, negative birth stories, that are shared with pregnant women and people are interesting to me. It's clear from the perspective of the media that drama sells. So to create stories around those who have calm, positive, relaxed births where they breathe their baby down is simply not as exciting as those who punch, kick, swear and create the 'on the edge' illusion of 'will she/they actually be able to go through with this?' But when it comes to us recounting our tales, I don't think it's a lot more complex than just assuming we also just love the drama. While I know from surveying Calm Birth School fans and students that those with positive birth stories feel like they stand alone in a sea of negative ones, there's a sense of not wanting to be 'that' person who recounts taking labour and birth in their stride. So, instead of speaking up, they just keep their heads down.

I also think there is a sense of camaraderie around shared pain. And unfortunately, for many who haven't experienced a positive birth, sharing their story acts as a warning and sometimes feels like part of their healing. I think if you can relate to this, one of the best things you can do is to speak with a trained professional to get a comprehensive debrief on your birth story. Asking your hospital or birth centre to talk through your birth notes can often be a great step towards healing. And for those who recognize that they have experienced some aspect of trauma, working with a doula, hypnotherapist or even a counsellor specifically trained in helping women who have experienced birth trauma can be the missing link to moving beyond painful, negative memories.

— Tip —

If someone tries to tell you their birthing horror story, you have my express permission (actually, this is an order!) to get friendly with your inner child, put your hands over your ears and sing the 'La, la, la, I'm not listening' song. If that isn't quite appropriate, stop the conversation politely and firmly tell the storyteller you would prefer to catch up with their birthing story after you've had your own experience. You'll feel great once you have set a clear boundary and you won't be adding any negative stories to your mental database. If you find setting boundaries challenging, this is a great opportunity for you to start to tap into that protective maternal energy and use it to take care of yourself and your baby.

Without the appropriate counselling, hearing – or watching – other people's birth stories may cause a pregnant woman or person to experience a negative charge of emotion, which they then file into their brain's 'unsafe' database. Should they then be faced with a similar situation (i.e. going into labour), the subconscious mind may try to protect them from having the baby by releasing hormones that activate the survival mode – the fight–flight–freeze response that we discussed in Chapter 1 (*see page 9*). In turn, this can impede their ability to birth calmly, comfortably and efficiently, as their subconscious attempts to protect/stop the 'unsafe' event from taking place. If you feel you need additional support in preparing for a subsequent birth due to a previous traumatic experience, please take a look at the resources section at the back of this book. TCBS also have many instructors who have undertaken Birth Trauma Competency Training so that they can gently guide you through their hypnobirthing course and support you in the best possible way (instructors who have undertaken this training are indicated by a badge next to their listing in the TCBS Instructor directory (www.thecalmbirthschool.com/instructor-directory/).

The part of the brain responsible for activating the fight–flight–freeze response sits in the oldest part of the human brain, the amygdala, which doesn't understand language or logic. It responds to situations based on imagery and feeling: what we see, even if only in our imaginations, and how we feel at a particular time.

It is interesting that the body's hormonal and physical responses are incredibly similar, whether we are seeing an event for real, imagining it or dreaming about it. This is why your skin feels damp from sweat and you experience an increased heart rate when having a nightmare. Even though you're dreaming, the brain can't tell the difference between what is real and what is imagined. It responds to what you're seeing and feeling in your dream in the same way as though you were having the experience in real life. Let me reiterate: the brain can't distinguish what is real from what is unreal. If you perceive an event to be 'true', either through your eyes or through your imagination, the brain will process that event as though it is actually happening and your body will respond accordingly.

In order to change the physiological chain of events that occur when you have decided – either consciously or subconsciously – that birth is unsafe, you have to literally retrain your brain to expect something different.

A simple process to help you retrain your brain is imagining or visualizing your ideal birth scenario and listening regularly to new audio input, such as audio download meditations. This simple process is so powerful because it enables you to begin to create a whole database of new 'memories' about how positive your birth is going to be, meaning you can change which category your 'birth' files are stored in, moving them from being labelled as unsafe and scary to being safe and positive.

I know if you're a first-time birther you might be thinking, 'Yeah, but I've got no idea where to start. I've never done this before.' However, a great resource for helping you with this is YouTube. Type 'hypnobirth' into the search bar and you'll be presented with some great examples of people birthing calmly and positively. My personal favourite is 'Daisy's Hypnobirth Homebirth' with mama Susy O'Hare. I love how calm, confident and in control Susy is, and how gently she welcomes baby Daisy into the world. Look for new YouTube inspiration once a week and you'll be off to a flying start.

Watching positive hypnobirthing videos regularly serves two purposes:

1. It gives you a real and tangible frame of reference that you can use to start building your own new blueprint for what birth can be like.

2. You can start to think about the different stages of labour and birth you'll experience and, if you particularly like what you see, mentally superimpose yourself into the films. Or think about how you would like to do things differently.

Create a positive birth story

In the following practice, I want you to start thinking about exactly how you'd like to give birth. But when you think or write down your birth story use the past tense, as though it has already happened.

Why should you write your story out in the past tense? A simple way to think about how the brain works is that it is a problem solver. If we ask ourselves a question, our brain will always look for the answer. By writing out your birth story in the past tense, you close the 'question–answer' loop in advance. I'll explain more about why this is important to you and your baby when we discuss the role of visualization during your birth in a later chapter.

How to do it

Use the following questions to help you start thinking about what you want to see, hear and feel during labour:

* Your blueprint or story may start with how you felt when you woke up in the morning, or at night with those first few cramps. How did you feel? Calm? Excited? Happy?

* What was the conversation like between you and your birth partner? Were they there with you? Or did you have to call them to let them know that you thought things had started?

* What did you do next?

* Did you go for a walk?

* Did you prepare some food?

* Did you watch TV?

* How did your body feel as your labour progressed?

* What rooms/buildings were you in?

* What did the room look like?

* Who was there with you?

* What did your body feel like when baby's head began to emerge?

If you find this too difficult to write out now, don't worry. Bookmark this page and write out your story once you have completed the book, if writing is useful. Or just start the daydreaming/visualizing about the day you'll meet your precious one.

When to do it

Once you have your ideal birth scenario in mind, daydream/visualize this story as frequently as possible; you can't think about it too often. When you're in the car, any 'dead time' you get at home, or when you're travelling to work, just start thinking and feeling into how you're going to be. The sooner you start creating this positive visualization, the sooner you'll start creating those new neural pathways for your brain to follow once the time is right.

· · · · · · · · · · · · · · · ·

You might have read through the above practice and may now be thinking, but I'm not a visual person!

Don't worry, I'm not visual at all, which is why I have you covered.

Perhaps you're more of an auditory person who loves to listen. In this case, working your way through the audio downloads that accompany this book (available for purchase via the website www.thecalmbirthschool.com/shop/), you'll really be able to embed the teachings by listening as you relax and even sleep. Although you might not have the visual pictures in your mind, the consistent repetition of the same positive approach to birth will create new blueprints for your brain to refer to when you go into labour.

If you're like me, and what they call a 'kinaesthetic learner', you'll probably learn best when you can move around and feel. So the way you can use this to your advantage when creating your 'visualization' is to think about how you want to feel during each stage. Imagine how relaxed the muscles in your face will feel if your surges intensify. Imagine your body feeling completely tension-free, like a rag doll. Maybe you'd even see yourself laughing and crying with joy once you are finally holding your baby. It's your birth: how do you want to feel? You decide.

✍ Wendy's birth story ✍

With my second child, I attended a hypnobirthing crash course with a TCBS Instructor, Karis. As a second-time mum, I wasn't really expecting to learn that much. I thought I had learnt all there was to learn. Boy, was I pleasantly surprised! I went in with a completely open mind, and let Karis work her magic. She covered so many topics, from hormones to affirmations, and by the end of the course I felt completely empowered and relaxed about what was to come. My second child also had to be induced (EDD+8)[11] but this time I was the one who made the call and I felt in control. I took the entire process at the pace that I felt comfortable with, and I only accepted the suggestions from the midwife that I wanted to accept. For instance, when they wanted to release my waters manually, I told them not to. And soon after, they released on their own! I remember being so relaxed during the surges that I was walking and dancing around the room while waiting for my cervix to dilate further.

My baby girl arrived five hours later, to a present, calm, and relaxed mama! It was such a beautiful experience, my husband and I both burst into tears of joy when she popped out! Thank you so much to Karis for helping turn my birth experience around and for teaching me the skills that resulted in such a wonderful birth!

CHAPTER 3

The Biology Bit

I hope you're now beginning to see how hypnobirthing is based in science – fist bumps all round. However, if you are still sceptical, this chapter will explain how staying calm and relaxed can have a positive physiological and emotional impact on your body and your ability to give birth the way you are designed.

The uterus and what happens in labour

No one knows why birthing women and people go into labour precisely when they do. If I knew the formula to that one, I'd be a very rich lady indeed! The most recent research tells us that labour begins when your baby is ready to breathe in the 'outside world'. While developing in the uterus, a baby will be receiving its oxygen from the placenta and its lungs will be developing in preparation for birth. Studies show that once a baby's lungs are mature enough they will release a protein (from their lungs) which will create a chemical reaction in the body and labour will begin in response to that. The body generates a huge surge in the hormone oxytocin which stimulates the muscles of the uterus and this kick-starts the surges.[12]

There are two types of muscle in the human body: voluntary, such as those in the arms and legs, which we can control consciously – and involuntary, such as the heart and uterus, which we can't.

The two layers of uterine muscles, one horizontal and one vertical, work together as a pair. They operate in the same way as any other muscle in the body, but you can't consciously move or control them. When you go into labour, the vertical layer of muscles moves down over the horizontal layer and begins to pull the horizontal layer upwards. When you're calm and relaxed, this movement is smooth – the muscles working together in harmony. The upward motion causes the neck of the cervix to thin and open so that the baby can move down the birth path easily, without stress.

You can see what this looks like here:

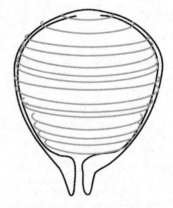

Figure 1: Inner layer of uterine muscle

The inner layer of the uterus is made up of circular horizontal muscles, which are located in the lower area of the uterus, with the thickest ones situated just above the opening or neck of the uterus (the cervix). For the baby to move easily down into the birth path, these thicker muscles must be drawn up and back.

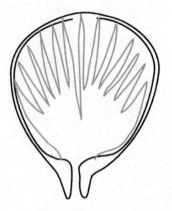

Figure 2: Outer layer of uterine muscle

The outer layer of the uterus is made up of stronger vertical muscles. These muscles go up the back and over the top of the uterus, drawing up the relaxed circular muscles of the inner layer.

When the birthing mother or person is in a state of relaxation, the two sets of muscles work in harmony in a wave-like motion. The vertical muscles draw up, flex and expel, and the inner circular muscles relax, open and draw back. Birthing then takes place smoothly and easily. Remember what we said earlier: your body is designed to give birth.

When you have a surge during labour, you may notice your tummy gets very tight and you can see things noticeably lifting, as shown by the dashed line in Figure 3 below. The uterus lifts as the muscles work during a surge and then return to their normal position.

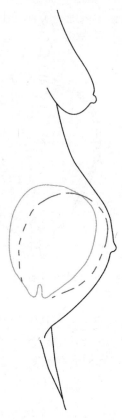

Figure 3: The uterus in surge

When you're tense or scared, the involuntary muscles of the uterus are prevented from working together in harmony. As the horizontal muscles tense up, the vertical muscles attempt to pull up these rigid, inflexible horizontal muscles. This state of muscular tension, along with your baby's head putting pressure on a cervix that isn't thinning or opening because of lack of movement, causes the pain that many people experience during labour. This experience confirms the initial fear that labour is indeed painful, which keeps you in a tense, stressed state.

Author of *What is the Size of Your Brain?*[13] Veronique Strohbach says: 'For every thought we have there is a corresponding physical and chemical reaction in the body.' Assuming we have healthy pregnant people and babies, this quote becomes the cornerstone of our understanding around how and why the uterus either works efficiently or becomes tense and inefficient when we are birthing.

In the previous chapter, I explained how the brain's database of memories sends messages to the body about what is happening (*see Chapter 2, page 24*). For some women and birthing people, another person's story will flash through their minds during labour, sending out a red alert that something is wrong. For others, something or someone within the birthing environment may trigger feelings of unease or being unsafe, which in turn puts the body into survival mode, as described in Chapter 1 (*see page 9*).

One of the body's key chemical responses to a conscious or subconscious thought of danger or threat is the release of adrenaline. Adrenaline isn't a friend of labour. When we go into survival mode, the physical response of the body is to divert blood and oxygen away from the uterus, because in evolutionary terms, the uterus would not have kept us safe from whatever the danger – real or perceived – was. As much blood and oxygen as possible is sent to our extremities because of their ability to help us fight for our lives (with our hands) or flee for our lives (with our feet). The uterus is understandably deemed useless and, as such, it is starved of the blood and oxygen it needs to function and becomes less and less efficient.

This is great if you're about to be attacked by a lion, but when it comes to labour, this isn't a good scenario: the lack of blood and oxygen available not only slows the process down, but also makes it more painful. The pain then reinforces the initial thoughts of fear, confirming there really is something to worry about. As labour slows and the birthing person becomes tired, they are much more likely to need some kind of intervention as their body, and baby, become less able to cope with the impact of the stress response.

In other words: fear equals tension equals pain.

— **Tip** —

Whenever you're feeling stressed, but particularly in the run-up to and during labour, one of the best things you can do to counteract the fight–flight–freeze response is to bring your attention to your breath and focus. The TCBS breathing technique you learned in Chapter 2 (*page 16*) will help to neutralize the stress response and create a release of endorphins.

Why endorphins are your new best friend

Endorphins are amazing for birth and a great friend of labour. They act in a similar way to opiates in the body and are said to be up to 200 times more effective than morphine when it comes to pain relief – which is why you ought to love them. The more things you can do to relax and feel good during the early stages of your labour, the more of those happy hormones you'll bank, helping you feel more at ease, more in control and more comfortable.

The other hormone I mentioned earlier, and one you need for an efficient labour, is oxytocin. Oxytocin is 'the hormone of love', a chemical we release into our bodies whenever we feel love for something or someone. When you make love to your partner, your body courses with oxytocin. (It's the reason many of you are reading this book with your lovely bump!) Oxytocin is the hormone that gets labour started. When you're able to stay feeling calm and at ease, it's also the hormone that causes some birthing women and people to feel euphoric and even joyful while birthing. The biggest peak of oxytocin arrives at the end of labour. This happens in between birthing baby and expelling the placenta (or afterbirth, as some people like to refer to it).

Oxytocin is the reason why, no matter how moulded, squished or messy baby's head will appear when they are born, many will look down into their newborn's eyes and fall totally and utterly in love at first sight.

This is part of nature's very clever evolutionary tool. It makes us want to stay close and look after our babies, which ensures the survival of the human race. The physiology of birth remains pretty much the same as it was over 200,000 years ago when homo sapiens first appeared. Not only did nature get the third stage right, birthing the placenta, but it also got the first and second stage, early labour and the birthing phase, pretty spot on too. Healthy women and people needed to be able to give birth as efficiently and as enjoyably as possible, because when we revisit what early human society looked like, there were no doctors, midwives or doulas (in the form that we know them, at least) at all. Yet birth happened again and again many times over, until we found ourselves here in the twenty-first century.

In short, we are designed to do this job. As you release resistance in the lead-up to giving birth and deepen your trust in the knowledge that your body and baby know what to do, when you reach your labour day, you really can let go and follow whichever direction your baby decides to take you in.

Pain

The time has come to put something on the table: we need to talk about pain. By now you should have a very clear understanding of the science behind why some will birth really comfortably, while others do not. As we mentioned a few moments ago there is a relationship between the kind of thoughts you think, the amount of fear you feel, how tense your body becomes because of that fear, and how much pain you experience. Once again:

Fear = Tension = Pain

Does this automatically mean that if you're fearless, you won't feel any pain? No: there are no hard-and-fast rules about how you'll experience the sensations in your body when you're giving birth.

Some of you reading this book will birth in complete and utter comfort, feeling relaxed and open, without resistance and able to birth your baby while feeling sensations but not pain. Others of you will feel sensations that you might have previously described as pain, but by preparing for your birth and mastering the techniques in this book, you'll feel that the experience is totally manageable. You'll find that you can distance yourself from the experience by using your TCBS techniques to keep you in the zone. Or you might also get to the other side of your labour and say, 'It was bloody painful, but I rocked it!'

Every experience is subjective and not something you can measure your own birth against. Whether you feel pain or not, whether you roar like a lioness or focus all of your energy inwards, giving birth will be your own unique journey. If you're birthing without fear, and feel able to surrender to whatever it is your body calls for you to do in the moment, you will more likely interpret your birth as a positive experience.

And be mindful that we all experience pain differently, depending on how we are feeling emotionally and what our brain decides is the most important focus in any given moment. If you have bad period pains but a lot of work to do, you're more likely to power through things, focusing on the task at hand rather than worrying about how your abdomen feels. But the minute you finish your chores and sit down, the pain suddenly hits you. This is because you no longer have the distraction of your to-do list to focus on. This is why breathing techniques, visualizations and, for some people, audio downloads play such an important role in their births, as they become a distraction from the sensations of labour.

The key marker for those who do experience intense or painful births, but who also have the tools of hypnobirthing in their back pocket, is that they understand that whatever they are experiencing is totally normal and nothing to be fearful of. This allows them to redirect their focus and choose to experience the physical sensations in a different way.

— Tip —

One of my favourite affirmations, reinforcing the idea we can choose to feel the sensations of birth in whatever way we desire is:

'Each surge brings me closer to meeting my baby.'

You can see how thinking in that way makes the sensations far more appealing and something to be welcomed from that perspective.

If, when you're birthing, you think about what a nightmare everything is, when you are going to feel the next surge and for how long, the whole experience becomes tiring, draining and intense. So from here on in, if you haven't been doing so already, rather than focus on how painful labour is going to be, it will be much more helpful for you to be curious about which techniques are going to help you remain comfortable.

I also recommend that you explicitly ask anyone involved in your birth to talk about your comfort level, as opposed to how much pain you're in – more on this in Chapter 7, when we'll also address communicating with your care provider. Remember that when you're sat in a state of relaxed consciousness, you'll be far more open to suggestion; you don't want a well-meaning midwife making an indirect suggestion that you need assistance because you could be coping more effectively with the pain, and for you to start analysing that, taking her suggestions on board.

If you can look at the sensations within your body as part of the normal process of birth, feeling at ease with what you're experiencing and knowing you don't need to fight against it makes the whole process much easier. You're able to experience the intensity of birth without fear, knowing that the sensations you're feeling are normal and natural, and reminding yourself that all you have to do is allow your body to go with it. Release all resistance. The way you experience that intensity or pain becomes a wave that you're able to ride, rather than something you're trying to fight against, as Karis's story below demonstrates.

✍ **Karis's birth story** ✍

At 41+3 weeks I relented and agreed to a sweep,[14] having refused one the week before. We made the decision, with the help of TCBS, that a sweep was really OK and might help things move on a bit. My parents had come over from the UK for one of the guess dates and I was feeling the need to get a wriggle on (not that there was any pressure from them; it was my perception).

We were getting the endorphins going left, right and centre. I was still riding my bike and going for walks; my parents even went out, saying to us, 'Go on, have vigorous sex!' (Not what you want to hear from your churchgoing mum.) I even went for a jog!

The sweep didn't work but my blood pressure was high, so the midwife told us to call the hospital. After being monitored twice previously during the final month, I was told it wasn't high enough to worry about, so off we went back home. After supper that evening, I felt strange and knew something wasn't right. I took my blood pressure again and it was much higher than before, so back we went to see the midwife and this time we were sent straight to hospital.

My plan to labour at home and have a water birth was off the table, as after 41 weeks you're no longer under midwife care. I was monitored overnight. My blood pressure remained high but stable. My mum has had a brain haemorrhage, so we didn't want to ignore the high BP (blood pressure), and I was happy that baby and I were being monitored.

In the morning, I was given a Foley catheter[15] to encourage my cervix to move and start to dilate. Was it invasive? Possibly, but I should say that having read the statistics I knew that my baby was not coming out naturally, and my TCBS breathing and affirmations helped me through the procedure. But I was also confident that the birth of our baby would be great whatever happened. After living with polycystic ovary syndrome (PCOS), we didn't think we would even be able to have a baby, so the end result was going to be worth it, regardless of the process.

That night Matt went home for some sleep (lucky him) and then the surges started. The catheter was doing something, at least. By 2 a.m. a giant Dutch midwife with the longest fingers ever came to see me and check on my progress. My cervix was still being backward in coming forward, but she could at least touch the membranes. Sweep done, catheter removed: time for me to get rest.

The next morning, with Matt back by my side, the doctors decided an induction was required, as my BP wasn't improving, and they wanted baby out.

Once in the birthing suite, I was hooked up to monitors to check my BP and the baby's heart rate, but I could still move around a bit, sitting, standing, squatting. Then labour began in earnest. I wasn't prepared for the strength of the hormone-induced surges, nor was I aware that there would be no let-up or break between them. My first thought, What the heck?! *was followed by Suzy's voice in my head:* Breathe, breathe, breathe. *I had affirmations running through my mind the whole time, and at one point Metallica's 'Enter the Sandman' started blaring out, with Matt beaming at me. We were having such a good time. No, it wasn't what we'd planned, but we were going to meet our baby boy or girl by the end of the day!*

At 6cm dilated I requested an epidural, thinking I would get a reprieve. I'm a potty-mouthed swearer, but through the entire process the one and only time I decided to swear was when the anaesthetist gave me the pre-epidural prick. I shouldn't really have called him a MoFo. First, he and his assistant were both hot, and second, I would be seeing him later. Oops!

The surges came thick and fast after that. I thought the epidural would help or stop the discomfort, but it just changed it. I got onto the bed and Matt held one of my hands palm open while I used my other hand to stroke the bed bar up and down in time with my counting. Anyone in Room 11 will have the shiniest bar on the bed! It was working; we were doing this and loving it.

The midwife came back into the room to examine me: 8cm, whoop whoop! However, baby's heart rate was not recovering well. They did a blood gas test on baby's head, and the results were right on the cusp of their preferred readings. The midwife and nurse started discussing something in Dutch. I said, 'You're preparing for a caesarean birth, aren't you?' They told me that they always like to be prepared. The second test was done, and the tempo shifted gears; it was clear that they wanted to get baby out. They knew what my birth wish had been, and we were so far away from it that they didn't want to tell me. I was absolutely fine with the change of plan; I even said, 'Brilliant. Let's go.' For us, it was all about the journey to meet our Boo Boos, who arrived at 8:12 p.m. on Friday 15 May covered in poop: a beautiful baby boy weighing 7lb 8oz – not the behemoth we had been told to expect.

William had arrived, our miracle – the baby we thought we would never have – on a day that was so happy, enjoyable and mind-blowing owing to the work we put in with TCBS. I want to say to anyone preparing to give birth that even if your birth wishes don't happen, you can be in control of yourself and your reactions to the unfolding situation.

∾

··

Wave breathing

··

Use wave breathing when you're experiencing a wave or surge.

How to do it

The central idea of wave breathing is to keep both the inhalation and the exhalation even. Breathe in through your nose for the count of seven and out through your mouth for seven.

The role of this breath is to work with the upward motion of the uterus as it rises (*see Figures 1–3, pages 32–34*), and then to send your breath down to your baby and your womb, while relaxing. Simple!

However, don't be fooled. To move instinctively into that space of deep breathing and relaxation when you experience a wave, you need to have practised it so often that it is second nature.

Please do not worry if you're unable to keep the breath even for a count of seven to start with. Work with whatever feels most comfortable for you. Perhaps start off counting to four and once that feels good extend it to five. The main point is to become comfortable slowing your breathing down and taking control of the flow. This will help you immeasurably during labour and birth.

When to do it

Aim to practise the wave-breathing technique every morning for five minutes. If that means setting your alarm five minutes earlier – do it. It's such a great way to start your day and will leave you feeling great as well as preparing you for your labour day, when you'll be using it during each surge you experience.

··

CHAPTER 4

Taking Control: Do the Work

As you can probably tell by now, we like to tell it as it is – no messing around. We've explained that hypnobirthing isn't a magic wand, but it is one of the best things you can do to give yourself a great foundation for making your birth as easy, comfortable and positive as possible. (Yes, we will keep repeating this over and over. We have to make sure the old fear-based message is well and truly erased!)

By the time you have finished reading this book, you'll have all the tools that have been shared with thousands of pregnant women and people around the world who have created amazing births, the kind they're happy to share with anyone who'll listen! However, reading the book and listening to the audio downloads isn't all there is for you to do. You have got some work to do in order for you to experience the type of positive birth you've been reading about. Actually, make that a lot of work. Yes, you get points for showing up and reading, but that is just the beginning. The time has come for us to make an agreement. This may or may not go against all your sensibilities, but it doesn't matter. Wherever you are right now, I ask that you suspend any and all beliefs springing from doubt about your ability to create a really positive birth.

What is a belief?

Essentially, a belief is a thought that we have repeated to ourselves so many times before that we have categorized it as 'real'. By repeating your thoughts about your ability to create a calm and positive birth experience tens, hundreds or even thousands of times, you start to form a new belief for your subconscious to follow. This is a hugely important part of your preparation for your birth, helping you to look forward to your birth feeling even more confident as you mentally rehearse your birthing experience and your ability to navigate all or any of the situations that may be presented to you with ease.

Remember the way the brain works? When you believe something to be true – even if it's not actually true (in this case, that birth is painful and difficult and it's only fun once I get to the end bit), the subconscious will do its very best to prove you right and prevent you from experiencing this unsafe event. In practice, this can take the shape of slowing down or even stopping your labour, as it tries to stop you from giving birth, in order to keep you safe. This is obviously not what you want to happen! If you're in labour, you want your baby to come out, not to stay in, and delaying this process usually results in more discomfort and medical intervention that might not otherwise be necessary.

We embed new ways of thinking and responding to situations through constant repetition of new actions or thoughts. Think back to when you learned to drive; when you first started learning, you didn't think there would ever be a time when you could have people talking to you from the back seat, while having the music on, while navigating a new city. Every ounce of concentration had to go into using your mirror-signal-manoeuvre process, and you had to practise again and again (and again).

If you don't know how to drive, perhaps you remember learning to ride a bike; it took a lot of practice before it became instinctive enough for you to ride with ease. The only way we can change our subconscious patterns of belief is to know that there is an alternative to our ingrained thought patterns.

The following exercise will help you rewrite any unhelpful beliefs you might have about giving birth.

Using affirmations to change beliefs

One of the easiest ways to change your thoughts and beliefs is to use affirmations to choose consciously the things you want to say to yourself: to change your internal dialogue. Affirmations are simple, powerful, positive statements that you repeat often so that they become your new narrative to how you're going to approach and experience your birth.

How to do it

Write out the following and then say it aloud, as often as you can:

* I know I can enjoy an amazing, positive birth. I will immerse myself in positive birth stories.

* I will imagine my positive birth with feeling. I will do my daily breathing exercises.

* This is important to me because [*complete this sentence*].

And once you have completed that exercise, I would like you to do the same with the following sentences:

* I am creating an amazing and positive birth.

* I am immersing myself in positive birth stories. I am imagining my positive birth with feeling.

* I am doing my daily breathing exercises.

* This is important to me because [*complete this sentence*].

Changing the sentences from 'I will' to 'I am' takes things out of the future into the present tense – giving you no excuses to hide, and letting your brain know that this is happening.

When to do it

Don't do this exercise later: do it now, even if it's on the back of an envelope. Don't just think about it. Actually write it down and say it out loud.

It doesn't matter if you feel silly saying these words. What's important is that you're fully invested and believe in your body and your baby's ability to do the job they were designed to do, and if repeating some affirmations out loud helps you with this, then it's 20 seconds well spent.

If you're already feeling confident, relaxed and committed, this is a worthwhile exercise in reminding yourself why it's important to you to create a positive experience. It's a win-win either way. If, however, you're feeling a bit anxious and awkward, now is the time to leave Ms Cynical at the door.

Embedding your new thought patterns

You can turbo-charge the process of embedding these new thought patterns in your mind by adding emotion. Imagining how you're going to FEEL when you look at your baby in the eyes for the first time. Imagining how you're going to FEEL as those first proper surges kick in, and what it will feel like to have your birth partner observing you in all your strength as you calmly and confidently guide your baby out into the world. Play around with words, sentences and images if you can – just like I described with the visualization exercises – and get feeling!

So, how can we help you achieve this? First things first: if you haven't yet said the above affirmations out loud, stop reading right now and recite them. This simple act is symbolic: you're sticking your marker in the sand and declaring, 'I'm taking control now.' As you move through the course, you'll also learn how to let go of everything you can't control.

Here are the statements again. If you read them before, here's another opportunity to do it again and feel it:

* I am creating an amazing and positive birth.

* I am immersing myself in positive birth stories. I am imagining my positive birth with feeling.

* I am doing my daily breathing exercises.

* This is important to me because [*complete this sentence*].

Once you've declared this – and meant it, you might like to start listening to TCBS course of daily of affirmations. There are written versions available for free at www.thecalmbirthschool.com/bookbonuses or check out my prompts on the TCBS Facebook page. Start reading and reciting them every day.

If you're feeling sceptical of the 'war cry' above, I strongly suggest that you make time to write out and say the above 'I am' affirmations every day at least 10 times, before you listen to the recorded affirmations. Continue to practise the affirmations daily until you really believe them, then you'll be able to dive straight into the recorded affirmations without any preparation.

For some of you the words will resonate and hit home right away; for others, it won't feel real until the day you go into labour. Neither is better or worse. All you have to do is commit to getting there.

Once you've listened to your affirmations, decide which three or four you love the most. Write them down and post them around the house, on places like the bathroom mirror or the back of the front door so you're continuously reminded of the calm and positive birth you're creating.

. . . .

Dealing with worry and anxiety

Pregnancy and the thought of birth can take some of us by surprise. We can be so confident in other areas of life, but when it comes to our pregnancy bump, we get 'worryitis'. If you're already prone to worrying, the unknowns of pregnancy can simply add to your current anxiety. This isn't bad or wrong, and I've seen it many, many times before, so if you fall into this category, please do not beat yourself up for it but do use the exercise below.

. . . .
Release and let go
. . . .

The following technique will help you put those worrisome thoughts to bed so that you feel as chilled, relaxed and happy as possible, instead of tense, uptight and nervous. And the great news is that because worrying is simply a habit you have learned over the years, anything that can be learned can also be unlearned. Sometimes it takes a bit of practice, particularly in the beginning when it often feels easier to do what you have always done – which in this case is let yourself worry – but you have choices available and it's time to take charge.

How to do it

1. If you notice yourself getting into a worry loop, simply recognize it. When you do recognize it, don't beat yourself up.

Acknowledge what you're doing and try to laugh at yourself and lighten everything up. You can even say to yourself, 'Look at me, I'm doing it again!' This is important because by noticing and light-heartedly commenting on what's happening, you immediately interrupt the autopilot loop.

2. Once you have become aware of the worry, ask yourself, 'Do I want to feel worried/anxious/angry [*or whatever the feeling that goes with the worry*] or do I want to feel better?' Sometimes you won't actually want to feel better right away. I'm sure you can remember a time when a partner or a friend has annoyed you and you felt completely justified in staying in a mood with them, because you were not quite ready to move on from your worry or frustration. If this is you, that's fine, but remember to ask yourself the above question, as it will put you back in control of your process rather than at the mercy of it. Acknowledging that you're choosing to stay in the less positive space is the first step in truly moving beyond it.

3. If and when you do make the decision to feel better, release the thought and think about something that makes you smile, such as something or someone you appreciate or that makes you feel a little better. You could imagine lying in a lovely warm bed, or if you're being kept awake during the night, perhaps you could think about how great it feels to be on a beach with the sun on your face. For some of us, thinking about a lovely piece of chocolate, or a nice memory, or someone we love will do the trick. Once you have found your 'sweet spot', keep reaching for a better feeling or thought, until you're able to sustain that good feeling.

You don't have to go from feeling terrible to feeling amazing for this to work. Any slight improvement in your mood or distraction from your worry even for a short period is a win. And as with everything, the more you do it, the easier and more instinctive it becomes.

When to do it

Use this technique whenever you notice an anxious or worried thought. The first few times you try this technique, your mind will keep bouncing back to the negative place and the whole concept may feel disjointed. However, success comes with continuing to choose to focus your attention on a more positive thought – which works most effectively when the new thoughts are completely unrelated to babies, pregnancy or giving birth. Although this isn't easy, it's worth it.

This exercise is like any other workout: it takes time to get your positivity muscle working harder than the automatic 'Negative Nelly', who is so used to their job that they can do it without thinking. Once you've got it though, what you'll notice is that by practising regularly and reaching for a more positive feeling, you'll instinctively become more positive about your birth and life in general.

To sum up, your new three-step process to move from worry to chill is, in the following order:

1. Acknowledge.

2. Release.

3. Reach for a thought that makes you feel better.

CHAPTER 5

Creating a Positive Birth Environment

Now that we've covered a lot of the psychological groundwork for creating an empowering attitude towards pregnancy and birth, let's turn to the more practical details.

Choosing where you're going to give birth will hopefully be a fun and interesting process. I encourage you to weigh up the pros and cons of all your options. This chapter will guide you through the various choices available to you, and will empower you to find the best solution for you.

You might instinctively know that bringing your baby into the world at home feels like the most natural option – and then again, you might read that sentence and think, *You have got to be joking!* The beauty of The Calm Birth School approach is that there is no right or wrong place to meet your baby for the first time. The most important thing is, in the words of the amazing childbirth educator Sarah Buckley, that you feel 'private, safe and unobserved'. When you look at the theory behind that, it all makes perfect sense.

The cocktail of hormones generated when a birthing woman or person goes into labour are the same as those created during lovemaking. Can you imagine getting intimate with your partner and every five minutes having someone walk into the room and asking you in a loud voice if everything was OK so they could check your progress and give you a mark out of 10 with a clipboard in hand? Getting up close and personal with your vagina while making sure the very non-romantic strip lighting was turned up as high as possible? No? I thought not.

We also have to acknowledge we are mammals and there are certain common traits to any mammalian birth. If an animal is diurnal (awake in the daytime) they tend to go into labour at night, when things are quiet and the daily hustle and bustle is done. Have you ever seen a cat give birth? If so, you've been very lucky, because cats will typically search out the quietest place in the house so that they are unlikely to be disturbed. You might also notice that a number of the birth stories throughout this book are from people whose labour either started or took place during the night.

Our genetic make-up means we are programmed to want exactly the same thing. However, few of the more commonly used birthing environments in the modern Western world offer us a space where we feel a sense of privacy or even quietness. Think of it this way: if you wouldn't want to make love there, your body isn't going to vibe when birthing there without taking a few simple, but effective actions to make your space your own. I'll get to that in a moment.

First things first. In order to create a positive birth environment wherever you're choosing to birth, I recommend the following four-step process:

Step 1: Know your options

The options that are available to you will depend on local medical facilities or whether you're prepared to travel to a particular hospital or birthing unit. However, most birthing women and people can choose from the four birth scenarios:

1. Home birth

If you're enjoying a low-risk pregnancy and all the signs indicate that your baby is healthy and happy, you may opt for a home birth. NICE (the National Institute for Health and Care Excellence in the UK) has stated that for second-time mums, home births or low-tech, midwife-led units provide better birth outcomes in terms of safety and lower rates of intervention than hospital births. A study published in April 2020 found that people who intended to birth at home as opposed to hospital were less likely to experience intervention, including caesarean birth and operative vaginal birth. They were also less likely to require the use of an epidural, an episiotomy, or oxytocin-augmentation of labour, as well as less likely to experience third- and fourth-degree tears, maternal infection or postpartum haemorrhage.[16] In fact, in the UK it is your legal right to birth at home, whether you're low-risk or not, and whether you have had a baby before, or not. Obviously, the decision about your place of birth should be based on an informed choice, where the risks versus the benefits have been weighed up.[17] In the USA around 1 per cent of all birthing people[18] choose to have a home birth, but that figure is steadily increasing. However, not all US states provide home births under their insurance-led healthcare system.

In attendance you'll have a community midwife, who you may or may not have met before; a caseload midwife, who you'll have grown very familiar with during visits throughout your pregnancy; or a private midwife (more likely outside the UK). Being in your own environment with a familiar care provider helps to promote the optimal environment for giving birth.

2. Birth centre

Birth centres are run by midwives and aim to create the same type of feeling or environment as being in your own home, or even better, a spa. The main difference between a birth centre and a midwife-led unit is that they often stand alone, i.e. not connected to a hospital. Often these establishments will have their own policies and ideas about who can and can't birth there (usually depending upon the type of pregnancy a person is experiencing). If you're based in the UK, there are both private and NHS-run birthing centres available at the time of writing. If you're based in the USA, many birth centres are currently covered by medical insurance.[19]

3. Hospital midwife-led unit

For many low-risk pregnancies, this is the middle ground between a birth centre and the labour and delivery ward. This choice offers a place where midwives are familiar with physiological births and understand that you're looking for labour to progress at its own pace, with the knowledge the hospital is close by. Often this can be the ultimate reassurance for someone, helping them to feel at ease should special circumstances arise.

4. Labour and delivery unit

A traditional hospital birth is usually the number-one option for birthing women and people who have health issues or are experiencing more complicated pregnancies. If your labour and birth progress without issue, your care will be predominately midwife-led. But the labour ward offers consultant/obstetric-led care. Should you request stronger pain relief, such as pethidine or an epidural, then generally speaking, these drugs can and will be administered here.

In the USA, many hospitals offer family-centred care: private rooms where you can go through labour, delivery, and recovery all in the same room. After birth, your baby stays in your room with you.[20]

➷ Jenny's birth story ➷

On Saturday, 3 April I started to feel mild cramping... it was coming and going throughout the day. About 20 minutes apart, at varying lengths. I thought to myself, 'could this be the start of early labour?!' I went through the whole day and night feeling these mild cramps. Got ready for bed and went to sleep wondering if my time was coming soon. Then at about 2:30 a.m. on Sunday morning, 4 April, I was awoken by a very intense cramp. I thought, whoa! OK... now this feels like this could be for real. The cramps had definitely intensified into what I thought could be considered a mild contraction, or 'wave'. The time between each wave varied, from 20 minutes, to 7 minutes, to 15 minutes... It went on like that entire day on Sunday. I stayed active throughout the day, walking on the treadmill, bouncing on my exercise ball and practising my wave breathing each time I felt a sensation.

I was getting a little emotional, wondering when things would really kick in, and when I would go into 'active labour'. But I remembered to practise 'acceptance' and just live in the moment as it was happening. This allowed me to stay calm. I called triage around 5 p.m. Sunday night and described what was happening... they said it sounds like you're in the 'early labour' phase, and you need to stay home. So I did... In the meantime, I had experienced some spotting and the loss of my mucous plug. So I thought, OK – things have got to get happening now!

I felt waves all Sunday night. I stayed upright on the couch instead of lying down because that felt better, and I breathed through each sensation. Things continued the same way all day Monday, 5 April. The waves were starting to build in intensity and then finally, they started to get closer together in frequency. I continued walking on my treadmill and leaning on my partner and other furniture around my house! That really gave me some relief. I called triage again around 5 p.m. on Monday, 5 April and they told me to come in. They could tell that the hours of labour (about 30 hours now) at this point had really started to wear me out. I was getting quite tired, but I felt calm and focused throughout the entire process.

We arrived at triage, and I got my cervix checked by the midwife. I was 2cm dilated... But my blood pressure was elevated, and they said I appeared to be quite dehydrated. So they wanted to admit me to keep an eye on the situation. During this time, we went over our birth preferences and expressed our desire to have a 'tub room' and to have a vaginal delivery. I was admitted to a tub room and assigned a midwife. She discussed with me the option to get an IV of fluid to help rehydrate me and also some morphine to help me get some rest between waves to gain strength for the 'active labour' phase. We made the decision to move forward with the morphine and the IV.

Once I was given the morphine, I felt my whole body relax... after I lay on my left side hoping to get some rest... As I relaxed the waves started to build in intensity. After about an hour I asked the midwife if she could check me again because I felt the intensity had increased to a point where I wanted to know how dilated I was. She checked me and I was 7cm! Oh – and also my waters released as she was checking me! All of that progress in just one hour! So she said it was time to start filling up the tub. Once in the tub, the relief I felt was so amazing! We had turned out the lights and I was able to just focus on the sensations and use my breath and my voice to get through each moment... I was in the tub for about an hour when I started to feel an intense 'bearing down' feeling... A feeling like I wanted to push. I asked the midwife to check me again, and I was 10cm... It was time to start pushing!

I remembered my breathing techniques I learned from class, and I started to 'breathe my baby down'... I could feel the progress of my baby moving down my birth path and she and I worked together with each push... At one point I found myself hesitating because I had some fear of what it would feel like to actually have her come out! But I thought – now is not the time to be afraid – now is the time to do this! So I abandoned any fear I had and just pushed with each sensation. After about 30 minutes, my baby girl was delivered in the tub and I was pulling her out of the water looking at her little face. I felt so much emotion! Relief, amazement, and shock! I couldn't believe I had actually done it! Something I had prepared for and anticipated for so long, my labour and delivery of my baby, and I had actually done it! The midwife said she couldn't believe how well I did for a first-time mom. She was so impressed with how well I worked with my body and remained calm. She was so excited to do a water birth! I know all the methods I learned from class got me through my 48-hour labour. I felt such a sense of achievement afterwards, I was so proud of myself and my husband. He was a huge source of support and strength for me throughout everything, thanks to the tools that he learned from class as well.

I look back on my story feeling pride, happiness, amazement and like I can do anything! I'm so grateful for the Calm Birth School, my instructor Katie and all the tools I have now to face anything that life brings me.

Step 2: Ask questions and investigate

Once you have a sense of where might be the right place to give birth, you can start investigating in more detail. It's vital to give yourself permission to ask questions. If, for example, a hospital labour and delivery ward feels like it might be the safest place for you to birth but you would like a physiological birth, I would advise you to:

- Look up the hospital's statistics for vaginal births versus unplanned/emergency caesarean births.

- Find out whether the hospital supports physiological labours and births.

- Investigate what their general policy is for a woman or birthing person who is on the borderline for gestational diabetes/obstetric cholestasis/pre-eclampsia (if relevant).

These are all important questions that, depending on the responses, will either make you feel reassured this is the right place to give birth, or not.

Step 3: Get to know your environment

If you're going to be birthing in an unfamiliar environment, ask to be shown around the unit. This helps to reassure your subconscious on the day that there is nothing wrong because you have been there before.

If you think about it, before getting pregnant, when would you be most likely to visit the hospital? When you were feeling sick or injured, or when someone else was sick or injured. This isn't exactly reassuring for your subconscious! Therefore, if you're choosing to birth in a hospital, getting familiar with the environment and the care providers during a time when you're feeling relaxed and confident signals to your subconscious that there's no need for you to either consciously or subconsciously be on high alert once the time comes for you to visit when you're in labour. In the era of the pandemic (COVID-19) this wasn't possible and so many people would rely on a virtual tour of their potential birthing unit.

Although this isn't ever going to replace physically seeing, smelling and sensing the place you're considering birthing in, it is a decent alternative. While it's completely normal for your labour to slow down when you move from your familiar home environment to the hospital or any new environment (in order for the subconscious to double-check there is no imminent danger in store), you can help lessen the impact if you get familiar with where the action is going to happen beforehand.

Step 4: Make it your own

We mentioned earlier that the most important things for you to feel are private, safe and unobserved (*see page 53*).

Regardless of where you plan to birth, you want to create an environment where you and your birth partner feel as private as possible and completely safe. I often have clients include a sign for the outside of their hospital-room door stating 'Hypnobirthing couple. Quiet please, and please knock before entering'.

While you might be cringing at the very thought of doing this, I urge you to put your concerns to one side and remember that you only get to do this once. So if a sign on the outside of the door is going to remind your care providers to speak in lowered tones and of the type of language you'd like them to use, then it is worth it (*see page xxv*). These seemingly small shifts are really important in helping you to create a birth experience where you feel calm, private and respected.

Think about your birthing environment as a kind of love or birthing nest. If you're birthing at home, what would be good to have on hand to make your experience as comfortable as possible? If you're birthing outside of the home, what can you take with you to help you feel relaxed and happy, bringing with it the familiarity of home? This is important because home will be the place where the vast majority of people will feel at their most safe, so recreating that sense of security wherever you're birthing can only serve you.

Here follow some ideas for making your birth place feel as comfortable and as homely as possible – make sure you include them in your list and let your birth partner know exactly what you want and need on the day (*more on this in Chapter 9*):

- fairy lights – always top of the list – and LED candles

- fluffy towels for post-birth (your birth facility will have towels, but if your thing is super-soft luxury, then this may be for you)

- pillows

- room spray/face mist

- pictures of loved ones

- iPhone or smartphone, bluetooth speaker and charger, iPad or other device to play music or audio downloads

- back-up battery pack or portable charger for phone, iPad, etc.

- handheld fan

- massage oils

- portable blackout blinds (also great for once your baby arrives).

Certain objects will trigger happy and comforting memories for you, so start noticing which items you can consciously and deliberately create positive associations with in your home environment that you can then take with you into the birthing room. Some of my clients create their own birthing playlist, which is a great idea. If you want to do this too, I recommend taking the time to listen to your playlist and practise your breathing techniques while listening before you go into labour. Listening to this out loud means that your baby will enjoy it too!

Others like to spray their rooms with their favourite scent. Lavender is very calming and soothing, and spraying it around your bedroom in the evening before listening to your audio downloads is a great idea. By the time you go into labour, you'll have a really strong association with your chosen scent, which you always smell when you're feeling relaxed and at ease.

CHAPTER 6

Choosing Your Care

Choosing who is going to support you as you welcome your baby into the world is an important part of your preparations. You want care providers who are going to make you feel special, cared for, understood and respected. Having these core needs met will contribute to how you feel on the day you give birth. The more at ease you feel with the people who are going to be supporting you, the more likely it is you'll be able to create a positive birthing experience.

Professional care

During all stages of care, including the day you give birth, it's important that you like and feel safe with the team you're working with. If you do not feel positive about your midwife, OB-GYN or consultant, you're entitled to ask for a different member of staff to work with at any stage.

Some people think it will be too embarrassing to ask for someone else, or don't want to be known as 'that difficult hypnobirthing couple'. They might worry that there won't be enough staff to accommodate their wishes. A phrase that has always served me well when working with my face-to-face clients is, 'What other people think of you is none of your business.' Certainly, when it comes to staffing, it's not your responsibility. The only thing you need to concern yourself with is feeling safe and comfortable, so you can feel positive during your pregnancy and, crucially, during your birth, where one of your primary tasks is to help your body to work efficiently. If a member of the care team causes you to feel tense, anxious or even angry, this can slow your labour down as your subconscious attempts to protect you and your baby from the perceived threat in your environment by triggering fight-flight-or-freeze mode, the consequences of which we covered in some detail earlier in the book.

The main point here is that you only get to do this once. So, what do you think is more important: putting up with support that is actually hindering the natural process of birth, because you don't feel at ease? Or ensuring that every single person in your space can serve you in the way that is going to be most conducive for you to enjoy the birth experience you desire?

Who will be in the room with you?

There's an old wives' tale that you can put an extra hour onto your birth for every person who's in the room. Now, while I don't think this is true, feeling private *is* important. However, rather than focusing on the number of people in the room, we're going to focus on how safe *you* feel.

What can you do to help yourself feel at ease? Simple: Have your dream team surrounding you.

Primary birth partner

Ideally, this is a person who knows you really well. They will have been supporting you throughout your pregnancy and you'll have worked through this book together, understanding the techniques and discussing what will be most helpful for you on the day.

Managing your birth environment is one of the key roles of the birth partner, which we'll cover in more detail in Chapter 9. In brief, when your birth partner is in tune with you, they can sense anything causing you to feel stressed. The best way for your birth partner to heighten their awareness of how you're feeling is by being present and paying close attention to you.

Part of the birth partner's job is to respond to the subtle, and sometimes not-so-subtle changes, in your body, noticing whether tension is creeping into your posture, or whether you have a clenched jaw or worry lines across your forehead. If a particular person is triggering these things, that person should be asked to adjust their behaviour or asked to leave your environment without question.

Some of my clients have a trigger word or sign to let the birth partner know they need to do something, whether it's a look, a wink or a completely out-of-context whisper of an agreed password. They know they are needed.

Your birth partner is also your advocate. They are by your side and on your side, and should be the first port of call when managing your environment, so you don't need to worry.

It's important you feel confident that your partner can do their job effectively, as in an ideal world it is best to be disengaged from your rational and logical-thinking mind during birth unless absolutely necessary. This is because the minute you feel the need to get involved with stage-managing your environment, the more likely it is for you to be unable to stay in the state of mind that provides you with both the emotional and physical capacity for calm that you need to birth more quickly and comfortably.

I have been asked before: 'But what happens if I need to be able to make a decision about my birth?' And the answer is: then, of course, you make the decision. Hypnobirthing doesn't mean that you lose the power of control or speech at any time. But for situations that don't fall into the 'special circumstances' bracket, rather than having people asking you questions that constantly put you back into left-brain, problem-solving mode, it would be great for you to be able to trust your primary birth partner to do that job on your behalf.

Doulas

I love doulas! Doulas help to build a pregnant woman or person's confidence and, as experts in childbirth, will help you to feel relaxed, more comfortable and safe, while barely having to say a word. They offer unconditional and consistent support to you and your birth partner, providing better physical and emotional birth outcomes for mum and baby. Doulas can also be of great help post-birth too. Be aware that most doulas specialize in either being a birth doula or a postnatal doula.

A report outlining the benefits of continuous care[21] – this is care from the same care professional throughout your pregnancy and birth – was pretty unequivocal in its findings:

- 31 per cent decrease in the use of synthetic oxytocin (used during induction)

- 28 per cent decrease in the risk of caesarean birth

- 12 per cent increase in the likelihood of a spontaneous vaginal birth

- 9 per cent decrease in the use of any medications for pain relief

- 14 per cent decrease in the risk of newborns being admitted to special care

- 34 per cent decrease in the risk of being dissatisfied with the birth experience.

Why is having continuous care so powerful? Because it makes you feel safe and secure. Unfortunately, midwives are often unable to give you the type of continuous support that would be ideal, as they are working with multiple people and have huge amounts of paperwork to fill out while you're birthing. More recent research in support of doulas also indicates that doulas improve equity and provide culturally responsive care. This is achieved when a woman or birthing person works with a doula from the same ethnic, linguistic or religious background.[22]

You might be wondering at this stage, 'But what about my partner?' A doula isn't there to replace your partner at any stage of your journey, but a doula is likely to have more experience in birth than your partner and has been trained to support you both. A doula will notice the slightest stresses and provide you with the reassurance that you're going to be just fine in a way that a birth partner may not be able to do quite as effectively.

I read an amazing analogy about a doula being like a Sherpa[23] and it really stuck with me. Imagine you're about to undertake climbing a beautiful, but challenging mountain with your partner. Of course, you want to have them there, experiencing every step of that climb with you, BUT you also want to have your Sherpa: someone who has climbed the mountain many, many times before, a guide that is tuned in to the changing winds, has tricks and tips up their sleeve for getting you past any tricky bits and has the confidence of experience that they are transmitting to you, via osmosis. Having your birth partner in the room with you, if you are both keen for that to happen, can be magical and nurturing for both of you. However, the statistics are clear: those who are supported by doulas (both with and without birth partners being present) often experience better birth outcomes.

If you can't afford a doula, don't be afraid to approach mentored doulas that are still earning their stripes and charge significantly less. Or approach doulas local to your area and ask whether they offer any concessions; you'll be surprised at how many do. Stay open to finding a great alternative that will support you for a significantly lower investment, because they are available.

If you know that you don't want a doula, fear not! Millions of birthing women and people give birth every year without doulas and have fantastic birth experiences. In fact, Liz has never had a doula and Suzy has used a doula once, out of her three births. So as always, tune in to what feels good and if a doula isn't what you feel you require, then it's all good.

Named, private or independent midwife

Some regions in the UK and USA offer a named midwife, which means many pregnant women and people can build a relationship with the same person throughout their pregnancy and birth. As the report I mentioned earlier showed, continuous care helps you feel calmer and more at ease during labour (*see page 66*).

Imagine the difference it makes to the subconscious, sitting down with the same midwife throughout your pregnancy. Having them get to know you and your family intimately, as well as all of your wishes and concerns. Knowing everything they need to know about you. How reassuring is that going to be? And if you're not birthing in a hospital, they will be the person who helps you to guide your baby out into the world. The peace of mind the right independent midwife can help to provide is, for many, priceless.

Mum/mother-in-law/sister/relative/best friend

While some of you may cringe at the thought of your mother-in-law being at your birth, for others it won't be out of the realms of possibility.

Neither is right or wrong. The only thing you need to consider is whether the people you're thinking about are up for the job. Are they able to put their own needs aside and put you and your beautiful new baby at the centre of their focus, while giving you the kind of support you most want and need? If you feel confident in having a family member or friend as your birth partner, then great. If you're not so sure, perhaps put them on the 'first to know when baby is here' list.

Holding the space

Whoever you choose to support you during your birth, the main job facing them is to 'hold the space' for you. They will best be able to do that if they feel prepared and calm and at least have an understanding of what you have been learning in your preparation. Inviting your birth partner to practise the breathing techniques isn't only for your benefit; it will be great for them too, helping them to stay calm and relaxed during your birth and ensuring they aren't sending out any subtle subconscious vibes to you that there's something to worry about.

CHAPTER 7

Communicating with Your Care Providers

One of the best things you can do to create a positive pregnancy and birth experience for you and baby is to make sure all the services and advice you receive are specific to you and your situation. This means asking questions of care providers in a way that provides you with very specific information to your unique pregnancy and birth, rather than accepting general rules of thumb that may not be applicable to you. This is important, both in the lead-up to birth and on the day.

It can be intimidating when a care provider tells you that you need to take a specific course of action, which you either don't understand or feel is unnecessary. Having the confidence to ask *why* and *how* certain things are relevant to your specific situation can make the difference between creating a positive experience and feeling like birth was something that 'happened to you'. I will share a specific set of questions you can use later in this chapter.

When you practise asking questions during pregnancy – such as 'What makes you think that about me in particular?' or 'What would best suit me in this situation?' – you'll gain clarity, which will allow you to make informed decisions about how you would like to progress. Having a sense of control is a key barometer for wellbeing. This need is particularly heightened during pregnancy and birth.

While sometimes you may conclude the best thing to do is relinquish control and move forward with your caregiver's advice or opinion, when that decision is made by you (armed with facts that are relevant and specific to your pregnancy), you remove doubt and confusion and know that the decisions you made enabled you to get the right birth for you and your baby on the day.

Use your BRAIN

In order to access an experience of feeling calm, empowered and in charge of your birth, I invite you to lead and direct the conversation using the acronym BRAIN to get clear on what is being requested or suggested by your care provider. You can then make your decisions in an informed way, and as a team.

B – Benefits

What are the benefits to me and my baby of moving forward with the suggested action?

R – Risks

What are the risks to me and my baby of moving forward? What are the risks of not moving forward?

A – Alternatives

What are my other options?

I – Instincts

What is my instinct on this, my gut feeling?

N – Nothing

What is the immediate risk if we choose to do nothing for the next 30/60 minutes? (Be specific about the time period.)

When it comes to your pregnancy and birth, clarity is king! So, remember to use your BRAIN and give yourself the opportunity to make informed choices.

— Tip —

It is also a good idea to include in your birth preferences that unless there is an immediate medical need for either you or your baby, you and your birth partner would like to be given the time and space needed to discuss your options.

Birth preferences

You'll communicate with your care providers via your birth preferences, commonly referred to as your 'birth plan'. I deliberately don't use that term when talking about your birth choices, as plans can often feel more definitive – and from the stories you've already read so far in the book, you'll know that nothing is definitive when it comes to birth!

Making plans for a wedding totally makes sense, as it would be completely inappropriate not to arrange all the details in advance rather than express preferences: 'If you don't have enough salmon for the wedding breakfast, don't worry, we'll have beef.' However, birth can't be neatly packaged up in the same way as a wedding can.

Be wary of veering too far in the opposite direction, however. While there are no guarantees in birth, the idea of not completing a birth plan at all because nothing ever goes to plan (a comment that I hear frequently) completely misses the point. We recommend that when you discuss your birth preferences with your birth partner, you take an A, B, C approach.

Think about what you would like to happen during a straightforward birth (Plan A), how you would like things to proceed if you need some assistance (Plan B), and how you would like to be supported should you end up in a situation where an unplanned caesarean birth is the best course of action (Plan C).

Taking this approach means that while it is important to spend your time and energy focusing on your ideal birth scenario, you have also taken into consideration the practical elements that may arise should you not have a straightforward delivery. This serves you, your birth partner and your baby far more powerfully from an emotional perspective when you're able to navigate the 'unexpected' from a place of preparation, rather than having to make knee-jerk decisions on the spot. And while you can never plan for every eventuality, understanding the importance of using your BRAIN will also help you immensely to turn difficult situations into infinitely more positive ones.

> ## — Tip —
>
> Always have spare copies of your birth preferences in case you misplace one or need additional copies for extra staff or staff changes. For ideas on what to include in your birth preferences, please visit www.thecalmbirthschool.com/bookbonuses to download our birth preferences planner.

Ashleigh's story below is an example of how even when birth unfolds in an unpredictable way, you can choose to feel calm, empowered and in charge.

✎ Ashleigh's birth story ✎

Having spent three years struggling with infertility we finally fell pregnant through IVF in June 2020.

The infertility journey teaches you to take each step as it comes so I had only focused on the 'getting pregnant' part and once we passed the 12-week milestone, I started to let myself think about the type of birth I wanted.

Hypnobirthing was a double win for me, as it taught me techniques I could use at birth but also tools to help with my pregnancy anxiety.

Our hypnobirthing sessions with our instructor, Jade, informed us about our choices for birth and enabled us to focus on what was important for us during labour and post birth.

Our sessions with Jade and reading hypnobirthing-focused books meant we had a clear birth preference but were also prepared and calm enough to go with the flow if things didn't 'go to plan' during labour.

With it being an IVF pregnancy the consultant was keen to induce us at 39 weeks. Being informed meant that we requested to wait, in the hope things would happen naturally.

In the end our little boy needed a nudge, and we were induced at 41 + 4 weeks. We felt much more comfortable with this choice and induction was likely to be more successful in leading to the calm birth we wanted.

The initial induction went smoothly and after 24 hours with the pessary I was ready to move to the labour ward and for my waters to be released. After a couple of hours and not much happening we opted for the oxytocin drip.

The labour started progressing and using my breathing techniques I was able to get through increasing contractions with no pain relief (much to my husband's upset as he was keen to secretly try the gas and air!).

All the signs of a progressing labour were there, and I requested that the midwife did not measure my dilation unless necessary. However, after 10 hours the doctor suggested that if things didn't soon start progressing more quickly, an emergency caesarean would be recommended.

A caesarean was our last preference for birth and, although a bit of a shock, we started talking about our options with the midwife.

Our midwife was amazing and recommended we give it two more hours (12 hours is the longest doctors recommend being on the oxytocin drip) and we spent the time going through our birth preferences to establish what was still possible with a caesarean birth. For example, skin-to-skin, delayed cord clamping and a calm environment.

After the two hours and little progress the doctor returned, and we made the decision to go ahead with the caesarean.

The whole medical team were wonderful and explained everything in detail before we headed to theatre.

People often talk about an emergency caesarean as a panicked situation and very dramatic, but I can honestly say that with the hypnobirthing techniques and going into the process really informed I felt calm and prepared to meet our little boy.

Everything went really quickly and before I knew it our little boy was being held up above the curtain in front of me. My husband cut the cord and he was then brought over to me for skin-to-skin. That moment is pure magic, and I do not feel I missed out at all in the feeling of 'birthing' my little boy.

Unless a caesarean is your choice there is no denying it can feel scary, but using hypnobirthing techniques and reading about your birthing rights you can still have the birth you want.

CHAPTER 8

Are Pregnancy and Birth Safe?

Trigger warning – safety in birth, race as a factor in birth and maternal mortality rates are discussed within this chapter.

Before we go any further, I want to reassure you that YES... birth is generally VERY safe.[24–25] There are studies and evidence to back this up. In the UK, for example, maternal mortality occurs in fewer than one in 10,000 pregnancies. Birth is safer today in the UK (in 2021) than it was 10 years ago.[26]

As we have explored all the way through this book, your body IS designed to birth your baby. Please keep that in mind as we explore the topic in this chapter.

It might seem odd, in a hypnobirthing book, to be discussing the safety of birth, something that could potentially create some fear, but we at The Calm Birth School aren't here for toxic positivity. We want you to have all the information you need to have a safe and transformative experience when it comes to the birth of your child and sometimes that involves discussing uncomfortable topics.

So yes, birth IS safe. However, there are caveats to this. Which means that, depending on factors like where a pregnant woman or person is in the world and what their race is, the outcomes in pregnancy, childbirth and the period beyond that can vary.

— Tip —

While we explore this further, you might not feel ready to read it or be triggered by part of what we have to tell you. So, anytime you feel you need to step back then please do so by taking some time to do The Calm Birth School breathing technique (in for four and out for seven) which will help you to feel calmer and process the information more easily.

High-income countries like Germany, Sweden, Australia, the UK and Canada (to name a few) are very successful, in general, at ensuring childbearing women and people are safe and well cared for.[27] This doesn't mean there isn't progress to be made, or that those countries aren't getting anything wrong.

It is interesting to note that all these countries have integrated midwife-led care into their healthcare systems and in all cases the number of midwives outweigh the number of obstetric doctors (or OB-GYNs). The WHO (World Health Organization) is among the organizations that have highlighted a need for more midwives on a global scale and has committed to improving the quality of midwifery education to ensure safer practice.[28]

The USA tells a slightly different story and in comparison to the developed and high-income countries mentioned above, it has the least success in maintaining good outcomes when it comes to pregnancy, birth and the postnatal period. However, bear in mind that poor outcomes are still considered low, especially when compared with developing countries.[29] Many factors contribute to these statistics in the USA, including too few maternity care providers, especially midwives, and lack of access to comprehensive postpartum support.[30]

The CDC (Centers for Disease Control and Prevention – the US health protection agency) is working to improve this situation and has taken action, including: continuing surveillance, statistical reviews and creating collaborations for the improvement of the quality of care received by mothers, birthing people and babies.[31]

What can you do with this news?

I firmly believe that knowledge is power. If you're in a country that needs to improve its safety record within maternity services (a little bit of research will tell you if you are), you're in a stronger position knowing that information, than not knowing it. Let's take stock of that... you're stronger WITH this knowledge than WITHOUT it. Now you have the POWER to plan around it.

Here are some things for you to consider, many of which we have mentioned before, but they become even more important now:

- If a hospital birth is the only option in your country or it is your preferred option, choose the right hospital for you. Do your research! Seek out a local professional (like a TCBS hypnobirthing instructor or a doula) who can give you a really clear picture of what care might be like in local hospitals. These are the people working regularly with women and birthing people who usually don't have a vested interest in any one type of birth or birthing place.

- Choose the right care providers! If obstetric care is the only or preferred option for you, find the right OB-GYN. You can prepare your birth companion to be the advocate that you need with the tools we discussed in Chapter 7.

- Could you explore a home birth? As discussed in Chapter 5, if available, this is a great option for some women or birthing people and generally speaking you would be cared for by a midwife in pregnancy, birth and beyond. As we have seen above, good, high-quality midwifery care (the standard of which does vary from country to country, so that is worth considering and investigating too), seems to play a key role in countries with good birth-safety track records.

- Are there birth centres available? Maybe you never considered this before, but for some people it is a fantastic option and, like a home birth, can actually lower your chances of intervention. The care is provided by midwives and the environment is often spa-like!

- Create comprehensive and well-researched birth preferences (*see Chapter* 7). Remember that the power isn't in the plans/preferences themselves, but in the actual process of creating them. Just by investigating or researching your options you create more understanding about how to create a safe, comfortable birth experience for yourself. You can more easily navigate any potential departures from your ideal scenario, your care team knows you mean business and you have peace of mind that you, your birth partner and your medical/care team know what you WANT.

- BRAIN, BRAIN, BRAIN (Benefits, Risks, Alternatives, Intuition, Nothing – *see page 74*). Don't forget this gem of a tool to help you navigate your options, challenges and choices in pregnancy, during birth and in the postnatal period too.

- Trust your body and the care providers you have chosen (when you have done all the above).

- All those tools, techniques and especially the mindset we have been cultivating throughout this book are absolutely VITAL to ensure you aren't stressed, and are able to navigate your birth experience as calmly as possible.

- Develop a plan for the postnatal period too (*we will explore this more in detail in Chapter 21*).

- Ask your care providers about what you can expect from your care in the postnatal period. (This is something many people forget to do or don't think to ask.) Know how often you'll be seen by a medical healthcare professional (and ensure that you can get to those appointments) and when you'll be discharged from their care.

- If you have any conditions that mean you have a higher chance of experiencing special circumstances, then as well as having an understanding of how this impacts your pregnancy and birth, ask about what a red flag for the period after having had your baby might be.

- Take care of your mental health. If you have experienced poor mental health before, consider what your potential triggers are, and if you don't have experience of this then please tell someone if you're concerned at any point. Share your thoughts and worries. Being a new parent is hard. It is OK to feel like it is too much – it is! Historically, in tribes and villages babies were cared for by a collective and the mother or birthing parent was also cared for too – we aren't meant to do this alone.

The Calm Birth School fear release exercise

Talking about safety in birth can be triggering for some people. This exercise is available to help you work through your thoughts and feelings (you can do this exercise multiple times throughout your pregnancy when you feel triggered or scared). Address your fears head-on and reduce the amount of fear and intensity you feel. This will help you to be as calm and relaxed as possible during your pregnancy and in the lead-up to the birth of your baby!

* Find a time when you can be alone (or not disturbed); turn off your phone and eliminate any distractions.

* Have a pen and paper handy. Now take a few deep breaths and ask yourself, 'What are my greatest fears?' Write down whatever comes to mind. There is no right or wrong answer. Nothing is too big or too small. It can be about pregnancy, birth, relationships, finances, work – anything that is causing you concern.

* Once you have written them all down, read over them. Do they all carry the same amount of concern or are some of

greater concern than others? Mark or asterisk the ones that cause you the greatest amount of anxiety.

* Notice how your body is responding when you're doing this exercise. If you're feeling anxious, focus on your breathing for a moment and take it slowly.

* Next, find a time (hopefully directly after you have written down all your fears) to talk through all the points of concern with your birthing partner, a close friend or family member. Make sure it is someone you trust.

* You'll find that by writing them down you can stop your fears from swimming around in your head. By talking about them you'll start to see if they are perceived fears or actual threats.

* Now, go and take some time to lie down and listen to your Fear Release audio download and let go of the intensity of those fears.

* Don't expect to have forgotten about the things that were really bothering you, but you should start to feel less concerned by them – more supported and with a renewed confidence in how you would deal with any of the situations that have brought you the anxiety in the first place.

* If you have some fears that you can't seem to reduce or begin to feel more comfortable with, speak to your care provider for reassurance and/or contact your hypnobirthing instructor if applicable (you can also post in The Calm Birth School Community Group on Facebook: www.facebook.com/groups/calmbirthschoolcommunity).

You can revisit this exercise again if you need to and you can listen to your Fear Release audio download whenever you want to.

. . . .

Does race affect my safety in birth?

The short answer to this, very sadly, is yes.

Why? Well although we know that the women and birthing people who have poor outcomes in pregnancy, childbirth or just after, can have multiple special circumstances, including mental health, general health, physical health problems and complex social factors, this isn't the full picture. Sadly, racism can also play a part in the safety of women and birthing people. More specifically, racial bias, institutionalized racism and systemic racism.

But before we get to the statistics and whys and wherefores, let's back it up a little.

Again, you might be reading this and thinking, *how odd to include such a triggering topic within a hypnobirthing book of all things?* And yes, we know that the topics of race, racism, disparities in health care and above all, the potential risk of mortality are all emotive subjects, especially when discussed in relation to pregnancy. But we can't sweep them under the carpet if talking about them openly might actually make a difference.

We approach this part of the chapter as a Black woman with lived experience of such and a white woman who aspires to be an ally.

If you aren't Black or Brown, Mixed Race or Asian, this chapter is still for you, because ultimately, it will take a joint effort, of all races, to make birth as safe for Black and Brown women and birthing people as it is for their white counterparts. You have your part to play – so please play it by first reading this chapter and then taking a look at the recommended anti-racism resources towards the back of this book.

— TCBS Suggestion —

If all those least likely to be affected by racism took steps to become anti-racist, think of the ripple effect that would have on future generations. Tackling racism in your own life (that means your OWN racism as well as challenging racist behaviours of others) is so important. That applies to all of us, even if you don't know a single non-white person. Even if you have Mixed-Race children or your best friend is Black. If you're Black or Brown yourself, the unequal power balance inherent in racism means you will be more likely to be on the receiving end of racism.

We recognize and acknowledge the particular harm racism causes Black and Brown people, and want to be effective allies in eliminating that harm whenever and wherever we can.

We recognize too that prejudice in all its forms is harmful. We all make assumptions, hold biases and carry out discriminatory behaviour – we all have a role to play in challenging it wherever it occurs.

To our Black, Brown, Mixed-Race and Asian readers, it is likely that you already know about the disparities we are going to discuss in a moment or, if you don't, it is likely that you won't be surprised but either way, this might be triggering for you. We suggest, as we did earlier, that you take this chapter slowly, put it aside if it feels too painful and return when you can.

We know that hypnobirthing isn't a magic wand, and it can't wave away or resolve a systemic issue like racism. Hypnobirthing is for everyone, and we intend to show you how you can use the tools and techniques that we provide at The Calm Birth School to help you to create the birth experience that you deserve.

So, let's get into some detail.

The research

MBRRACE-UK (Mothers and Babies: Reducing Risks through Audits and Confidential Enquiries) is a collaboration appointed by the Healthcare Quality Improvement Partnership (HQIP). In the 2018 and 2019 reports it was emphasized that the UK fares better than other countries in regards to safety in childbirth but it highlighted the alarming statistic that Black women, in the UK, are five times more likely to die as a result of special circumstances in their pregnancy than white women. And the 2020 MBRRACE report[32] identified that Black Women are four times more likely to die as a result of special circumstances in their pregnancy.

It is also important to note that it isn't just Black women and birthing people where this gap is experienced. For women and birthing people of mixed ethnicity, the risk is threefold and for Asian women it is double that of white women. (That has remained the same across all reports mentioned above.)[33]

While it is important to remember that, as discussed above, maternal mortality rates in birth are low across the board it is the disparities that are the major concern. The astounding statistics shocked birth workers like doulas, midwives, hypnobirthing instructors, etc., who are predominantly white, but to Black birth workers, Black mothers and people it was, unfortunately, not a surprise. Shock, particularly from white people, is useless. As Nova Reid (an author, TEDx speaker and anti-racism activist based in the UK) stated on her Instagram feed in 2020: *'All it does is highlight how unaware you are of the reality of racism in this country or that you've not been listening. It's painful.'*

A similar pattern occurs in the USA in regards to racial disparities. According to the Centers for Disease Control (CDC), Black and Indigenous Americans are two to three times as likely to die of pregnancy-related causes compared to white women in the USA.

So other than expressions of shock, despair and dismay, what is being done about it?

Despite the rise in disparity between Black maternal deaths and white maternal deaths being visible for many years[34] very little action appears to have been taken. In fact, it took until 2019 for any commitment to target the disparity when the NHS pledged to ensure that by 2024 three-quarters of pregnant Black, Asian and Minority Ethnic communities will receive care from the same midwife before, during and after they give birth. This target seems to be applied to those who need it most rather than as a blanket rule as such which isn't going to resolve the issue in its entirety because, as we learned a moment ago, there are many reasons why the disparity occurs (it doesn't just affect those categorized as being 'in need'). Professor Jacqueline Dunkley-Bent, OBE (Chief Midwifery Officer in England) stated 'Black, Asian and Minority Ethnic women will benefit where they are considered to be more likely at risk'. In fact, as highlighted by a Channel 4 *Dispatches* documentary in

2021, the Joint Committee on Human Rights stated in their report entitled 'Black people, racism and human rights' that the NHS '...*acknowledge and regret this disparity but have no target to end it'*.

It sounds pretty bleak, I know, but please keep in mind that the NHS is one of the safest systems in the world to give birth under, and there are few maternal deaths in the UK (it is the disparity that we are working to change here).

Let's look at the great work that is being done to raise awareness and ultimately create change

An amazing grassroots organization, formed in 2019 in the UK, called Five X More was set up by two Black mothers who had a goal and a vision to improve maternal mortality rates and healthcare outcomes for Black women in the UK. The co-founders Tinuke Awe and Clotilde Rebecca Abe have done ground-breaking work in campaigning for change and in empowering Black women to make informed choices and advocate for themselves throughout their pregnancies and births.[35]

In June 2020 the organization gained 187,519 signatures on a petition entitled 'Improve Maternal Mortality Rates and Health Care for Black Women in the U.K.' and parliament debated the petition on 19 April 2021. In reference to the absence of a target to end the disparities the then Minister of State (Patient Safety, Suicide Prevention and Mental Health), Ms Nadine Dorries MP, stated: '*We cannot set targets until we know what we are trying to achieve through those targets and what we need to address. Five X More has asked for that research to be done. It needs to be done, and it will be done.*'[36]

In the USA, organizations like Black Mamas Matter[37] are also working towards creating a world where Black pregnant people have the rights, respect and resources to thrive before, during and after pregnancy.

We hope in the very near future the UK and the US governments (along with other countries), the NHS and bodies like RCOG (Royal College of Obstetricians and Gynaecologists) and the CDC (Centers for Disease Control and Prevention) will have completed the research needed and are able to close the gap between maternal mortality rates.[38]

If you're a Black or Brown birthing person, how can hypnobirthing help?

Hypnobirthing aside, we would recommend you visit the Five X More website to read their 'six steps' as part of your preparation and to take a look at the other resources they offer there too.

As we said above, we know that hypnobirthing isn't a magic wand, but The Calm Birth School can teach you tools to help you navigate your unique experience of birth. We have listed some suggestions for you below to consider during pregnancy, in preparation for birth, during birth and postnatally too.

During pregnancy

It is widely reported by Black and Brown women and birthing people that many don't feel heard or listened to by medical professionals. Ease of communication is definitely a topic that needs addressing across communities and it has been said, in relation to poor outcomes, that if a woman or birthing person's care had been different, then their outcome might have been different too. We would recommend asking what the hospital anti-racism policy is and if staff have done any anti-racism training. In fact, at the time of writing, Five X More are in the process of piloting just such training with the intention of rolling it out across the UK.

From reading Chapters 5 and 6 you know that where you give birth and who you choose to be there are significant decisions to make. The care you receive is important, and if you aren't happy with the standard or level or care during your pregnancy, you can change it. You can change your midwife, your doctor, your place of birth – keep changing until you're happy.

As advised by Five X More, at each antenatal appointment take note of what is being said (or have someone with you who can do that for you). If you're advised to take a certain course of action in relation to your pregnancy and you choose to take that advice (it is always your choice) then ensure that it is written on your notes. If you request something (like a test or a scan or additional appointments) and it is refused, then ensure that the healthcare professional makes a note of that on your medical notes too.

In the UK it isn't illegal to audio or video record someone so you could do this in your appointments too. It is likely that the medical professional would protest at the recording, but they can't refuse you care and they do not have grounds to not 'allow' the recording. As Emma Ashworth (a birth rights activist) states on her Instagram feed, '*They are not allowed to refuse your consultation if you're recording because this would be a breach of their duty of care.*'[39]

Preparation for birth

As laid out in this book, it is important to prepare your mind from a subconscious and a conscious perspective as this will enable you to experience birth in a far more enjoyable way. As a Black or Brown woman or birthing person, you might feel an extra layer of fear when it comes to birth due to the information contained on the previous pages. With this in mind, although we would urge you to prepare as discussed, we have additional audio tracks available to support you through this.

Sabrina Taylor, TCBS Instructor, Cognitive Hypnotherapist, Mindset Coach and Black mother to three children has written some beautiful affirmations and a hypnosis track (entitled African Jade) exclusively for The Calm Birth School to inspire confidence, trust and intuition in Black women and birthing people. The tracks are available on our website and with each download a donation will be made to Five X More. I will include some of our favourite affirmations at the end of this chapter and some printable affirmations are available via our bonuses.

It is important while preparing for birth that, wherever possible, your birthing companion is able to be involved. As we discussed before, this will mean that they can be the best support and advocate that you need.

Choosing what you consume and absorb mentally during pregnancy becomes even more significant when considering the maternal mortality rates we have discussed here. As we will continue to reiterate, birth is generally very safe; it is the disparities we need to improve. It will help you to know that other Black women and birthing people have had wonderfully empowering, positive stories so immerse yourself in these. We have included a selection of birth stories from Black and Brown women from our community at the end of the chapter. You can also visit our YouTube channel to watch a collection of positive births which again will help you to recognize that you CAN experience birth safely and positively.

Revisiting regularly the Fear Release exercise listed on the previous pages will help you to navigate your fear or anxiety associated with the mortality rate disparity and asking for help or talking things through with a trusted person shouldn't be underestimated.

You may feel that this book and the audio downloads we have available via our website are enough to support your preparation or you may feel that you require something more tailored. If this is the case, I would recommend that you visit the instructor directory on The Calm Birth School website and contact an instructor who can work with you, either online or face to face in your local area. Many of our instructors have undertaken an additional workshop entitled 'First Steps to Anti-Racism' hosted by Black birth worker and founder of Black Mamas Birth Village, Lorna Phillip, and are committed to continuing their anti-racism education. Participation in the course is indicated by a badge/button on their directory listing.

During birth

By this point, ideally you'll have selected the best environment for you to birth in, you'll have chosen your care providers carefully and your birth companion will be fully prepped to support you. Although your birth partner is there to care for you, encourage you through the birthing process and undertake all the practical aspects related to birth, having a birth companion who is familiar with BRAINS (*see page 74*) and ensuring they have the confidence to speak up and advocate on your behalf is really important. You might want to consider an additional person as a support during birth who you feel would be able to focus on this aspect of your support. That might be a friend, parent or other relative, or you might opt for a doula (a skilled professional when it comes to advocacy and support in childbirth). As discussed previously, doulas actually improve many aspects of pregnancy and birth and they also have a positive impact on birthing people of colour.[40]

Abuela Doulas[41] are the UK's first Black-owned, -founded and -created doula course and you can find a doula via their directory. If that is something you're interested in pursuing, it is worth reiterating here that it is really important to interview doulas and find the right one for you. You need to be comfortable with everyone who enters your birthing space.

Utilize all the techniques included in this book to help you navigate your way through your birth experience. The mindset piece of the preparation with hypnobirthing comes before the birth and if you have committed to that, you're more likely to feel a sense of calm, confidence and empowerment as you navigate through the stages of labour. The breathing and relaxation techniques will help you to remain as chilled as possible, and allow you to work with your body. Lean into those who you have chosen to support you and feel their loving energy to help you to bring your baby into the world.

Postnatal period

As we said in the early part of this chapter, developing a plan for the postnatal period is vital and something we will focus on later in the book. Again, as stated earlier, ask your care providers about what you can expect from your care in the postnatal period and when you'll be discharged from their care. Understand if you have a higher chance of experiencing certain conditions and ask about what might be a cause for concern once you have had your baby. The same suggestions apply in the postnatal period, in terms of ensuring you're happy with the care that you and your baby are receiving, ensuring that you're documenting your appointments where possible, and that you have someone to advocate for you in those very hazy days of the postnatal period.

Remember to use your breathing and relaxation techniques to support you in remaining calm during this time, while you connect with your baby and recover from your pregnancy and birth experience. You can continue to use affirmations in the same way by utilizing our Mama or Parent Affirmation tracks.

Above all, throughout pregnancy, birth and the postnatal period, tune in to yourself, your instincts, trust the preparation you have done and trust your body and your baby. Remember for the vast majority of people, birth *is* safe. For those at higher risk, the information contained within this chapter will help make birth safer and more positive for you.

— **Tip** —

Affirmations for Black and Brown birthing people:

I am worthy of being honoured and appreciated.

I celebrate my uniqueness.

I love my beautiful melanin skin.

I love myself and my growing baby.

Birth Stories by Black and Brown women

Keep in mind that there are plenty of examples of positive birth experiences for Black and Brown women too.

∽ Gwen's First Birth ∽

Prodromal labour[42] was something I hadn't heard or read about in all my reading to prepare for the birth of my son. But it turned out to be how it all began: three consecutive mornings of being woken up at exactly 3 a.m. by sensations I'd call closer to extreme downward pressure than similar to period pains.

It then went to extreme pressure, which increased in intensity, getting me up and onto all fours holding onto the headboard of my bed each morning for two hours. And then just like clockwork, at 5 a.m. they stopped – completely stopped – and my partner and I would go back to sleep.

I was booked to be induced at exactly 40 weeks, which would have been the Monday afternoon. And so, on

Saturday night when my partner asked if he could join a friend's birthday bash I replied, 'Yes, of course! Just don't be too late back.'

As soon as he'd left the house on Saturday night I started doing all sorts of weird things. Things I didn't see as odd at the time... I thoroughly cleaned the kitchen, including the floors on my hands and knees. I locked up all the shutters in the flat, I sat down cross-legged on the floor and braided my hair into lots of little plaits and then sat in darkness in the living room for an hour or so.

Once it got to half past midnight, I decided it would be a good idea to get to bed and get some sleep. So in I climbed, expected to be woken up either by my partner coming home a little tipsy or by the now-normal 3 a.m. wake-up call.

It was the 3 a.m. wake-up call that did it. Only this time everything felt that much stronger. And I wasn't sure if that was because this time I was on my own (Daddy was still out, letting his hair down).

By 5 o'clock, the pressure wasn't subsiding as it would usually and so I sent a little message to Papa-to-be and urged him to come home and get some rest before we were booked to be induced on the following day!

Daddy was home by 5:40 a.m. and by then I knew this time wasn't practice. This was the start of the real deal. I felt excited! This was finally it!

I was still on all fours in bed and Daddy came in and attempted to get to sleep as we both believed we would be in it for the long haul – 24 hours or thereabouts is what we'd 'planned' to expect of labour.

So just after 6 o'clock, I got out of bed and ran the bath, walking a few laps of the flat while the tub filled up with warm water. I moved all my aromatherapy oils, oil burner and candles into the bathroom but by the time the bath had filled, the sensations had ramped up a notch or two and I ended up just hopping right into the bath with all the lights on, hoping to get myself more comfortable.

I sat upright with my legs crossed and my head rested on my arms leaning forward onto the side of the bath – I had just about enough room to bounce up and down in the water while still feeling relaxed and in an upright position.

And it worked, for about 20 minutes... at which point, I had to get out of the bath and SOS use the toilet. That's when Daddy woke up and walked into what may have looked like a disaster scene in the bathroom. Only I wasn't ill or hungover. With hindsight, I recognize I was transitioning from latent labour into active labour.

I got back into the bath while he cleaned up the mess. But it wasn't long before I began making some involuntary sounds that I can only describe as mooing and my partner decided it was time to call the hospital and just let them know things had started. The midwife on the phone asked him some questions and informed him that I was likely still in very early labour if I was able to talk through any pain. She invited us in for an 'examination', but indicated that we would be sent back home if it was found we weren't yet 4–6cm dilated.

Well, we really didn't want that. All the research had shown that travelling into hospital can slow labour down and so it's best to hold out and wait until you feel more sure surges are established.

Our plan? I'd take some paracetamol, get my breathing back on track and Daddy would start timing the surges, which I would still have described more as waves of extreme pressure than painful contractions.

I got out of the bath and did a few nude laps of the flat while my partner set up the birthing ball and a towel for me in the living room and a duvet for himself on the sofa!

Another 15 minutes of bouncing and circling my hips on the ball and I felt myself bearing downwards, which scared us both into calling our planned Uber ride to the hospital, and me throwing on some clothes.

Between the Uber journey and arriving onto the maternity ward, there was a lot of mooing and involuntary squatting on my part and a lot of very fast sobering up on Daddy's part!

We entered an observation room where a lovely midwife just starting her shift welcomed us and asked Daddy for the notes (we'd forgotten them). I unwittingly stripped naked and lay down on the stools set up for observations.

Our midwife offered me some gas and air to help with the surges and get me to stay still enough for her to find baby's heartbeat.

A few puffs later and she confirmed not only was everything fine, but I was also already 9cm dilated – definitely not moving to the labour ward (which was where we had planned to give birth) and certainly not going back home!

My waters burst pretty dramatically and actually I vividly remember how comforting a feeling the warm waters were... something I wouldn't have imagined from the expression 'waters breaking'.

A few short pushes later and our baby was born, just 20 minutes after arriving at the hospital. Safe and sound, he latched straight onto the boob and had an hour of perfect skin-to-skin time before getting some serious cuddle time from Daddy.

My first birth was the most AWESOME (and I mean awe-some), empowering, wonderful, surreal and magical experience of my life! It's made me a total birth junkie who's desperate to tell any women who are seeking an alternative viewpoint, that it is SO possible to have a POSITIVE experience of birth that will make you realize how you're PHYSICALLY AND MENTALLY built and capable of doing ANYTHING!

You can visit www.thecalmbirthschool.com/i-stood-and_moaned/ to read about the birth of Gwen's second child (a girl).

๛ Alyssia's birth story ๛

In the middle of the night, I felt mild cramping in my abdomen, prompting me to wake up and take a quick bathroom break (or so I thought). Rolling out of bed like a whale, I glanced at my swollen belly and whispered, 'Kristopher, I'm ready… I don't think I can do this any more.'

Slowly, I made my way to the bathroom and returned to my bed shortly afterwards. Within less than a minute, I jumped out of bed and felt a gush in my underwear. Upon proceeding back to the bathroom, I discovered the gush was my mucous plug… the bloody show! I returned to the bedroom for the third time in three minutes and stared at Brian, slightly envious of his deep sleep.

Shaking him awake, I said, 'Brian, things are moving along.' Lethargically, he nodded and went right back to sleep... lol.

I stayed up and proceeded with the routine that offered me familiarity and serenity. I opened the blinds, drank my daily cup of hot water with lemon, took some vitamins with my oatmeal and sat on my birthing ball in front of my computer, where I started to make bank calls and check my emails.

As I rocked on my birthing ball, I started to feel sporadic, light cramping, but found it to be super manageable.

I glanced towards the clock and made a mental note of the time: 9 a.m. I figured it was time to wake Brian up and prepare for our 11 a.m. appointment since it takes every bit of an hour to arrive in the city.

While he showered, I stayed moving. I gave the house a once over with some last-minute housekeeping and gathered our birth bags, as per my mother-in-law's recommendation. Earlier this week, my MIL (mother-in-law) suggested that we bring our birth bags during our visit in case they wanted to keep us in the city. Initially, I wasn't fond of loading up the car the day of our appointment, but, in hindsight, I'm so glad I did! Thanks, Patty!

With the car filled with our birthing bags, birth ball, yoga mat, vision board and more, we were ready to depart at around 10 a.m. You guessed it... we were running a little late!

Making my way to the passenger side of the car and bracing to open the door, I felt the cramping getting intense. I stood by the car door and focused on my breath until it passed. As I took my seat, I reminded myself: One cramp, one breath, one minute at a time. Brian suggested that we start to time the frequency of my cramps, starting at 10:18 a.m. The cramping came every six minutes and lasted 40 seconds to a minute until around 11 a.m. I put the timer away after 11 a.m. because I felt confident that things were moving along. I wanted to relax, prepare my mindset, and go with the flow.

How was I feeling during the car ride?

Good! I made sure to stay relaxed and breathe during the cramping sensations. Other than that, I remained calm and relatively 'normal', as I resumed my role of back-seat driver. Now, that's a norm in our family!

At 11:40, we arrived at the birthing centre for our 11 a.m. appointment. I immediately told the receptionist that I felt frequent cramping and signs of labour. In addition, I requested that both Brian and I take our COVID-19 test when she took me into triage to check my vitals, as I wanted to avoid wearing a mask while labouring. Props to all of the new moms who had their babies in a pandemic!

As she took my vitals, I felt two intense cramps that prompted me to stand up while my blood pressure was being measured, so that I could sway my hips back and forth and breathe through the sensations.

I started to give the midwife an update on how I was feeling. Immediately, she noticed I was in labour since I abruptly stopped talking with every surge. Oftentimes, I would raise my hand up, asking for silence, so that I could coax my body to relax and sway my hips back and forth.

The midwife proceeded to suggest a cervical exam to evaluate how far I was dilated, but I declined. For me, it was all about mindset to ensure a happy and healthy delivery. I did not want to know how far I was dilated in the event I was disappointed with the progress.

At this point, two senior midwives were invited into our appointment room, one of whom I knew well. We discussed why they wanted to move in this direction with the cervical exam and Brian demanded that I have one done, so I reluctantly agreed. The midwives also informed me that they needed to do twenty minutes of NST[43] testing on my stomach before I could be officially admitted, which I honestly was not too thrilled about. I was hyper-focused on my goal; all I wanted was to get settled in the birthing room to begin delivering Kristopher.

Once this was established, I requested the birthing room that I wanted to labour in and we proceeded into a temporary room while it was being prepared for us. It was in the temporary room that the cervical exam and NST were performed. I requested that the midwives refrain from telling me how far dilated I was.

In between surges, I would ask Brian to do some small things for me, like grabbing the birth ball from the car, plugging in my phone, or handing me my AirPods. As labour progressed, I was ready to zone out to my birth playlist and affirmations app.

The midwives hooked me up to the monitor and, 10 minutes later, they proceeded to tell me that the NST test was not producing the results they were hoping for and that the baby was in a 'sleeping' state. To stimulate the process, they advised me to eat foods like crackers or drink Gatorade to increase the chart readings. This was not what I wanted to hear, and I felt myself becoming frustrated and disappointed.

But, I knew what I had to do at this moment – and that was to focus on my baby and my more-than-capable body to deliver him. I chose to tell the midwife that I wanted all communication to be directed to Brian, as I wanted the spiritual, emotional, and intuitive part of my brain to reign supreme at this time. I felt confident in Brian – he knew what I wanted for our birth and took over, allowing me to focus inwards.

I paused to go to the restroom and told the midwife that I felt like I had to poop and she followed by asking if I had to push, to which I responded, 'Nope.' I went to the bathroom only to discover that I couldn't poop.

At this point, my cramps gained intensity and I started to feel super uncomfortable and hot, so I pulled off my dress and stripped down naked for maximum comfort.

Moments later, I noticed a few drops of blood on the bathroom floor. I didn't panic and I swiftly asked Brian to hand me a towel. When the midwife returned to the room, I told her about the bleeding and, to my satisfaction, she reassured me that nothing was wrong – I was just continuing to dilate. That's what we like to hear!

Eager to move things along, I followed their recommendations on eating and drinking and returned to the monitor to be evaluated for about fifteen minutes.

Outside of the room, Brian continued to communicate with the midwives as I handled the sensations inside my body – one cramp, one breath, one minute at a time.

Halfway through the NST test, the midwives collected the report and left the room. Moments later, Brian informed me that our birthing suite was ready – we were being admitted! Woo hoo! What a relief. It was time to get down to business and officially begin welcoming Baby Kristopher into the world.

Before walking to the room, I asked Brian if he would set up the room by closing the curtains, ensuring that the room was warm, and plugging in my phone.

I walked into our birthing suite and smiled to myself, as I finally realized that my desires and hopes for my birth were being manifested right in front of me. The room was perfect for the baby and me. Brian drew the curtains and the mood was set – I was able to get back into the zone and focus on what we came here for. Hopping back on the bed, I swayed my hips back and forth for a moment or two before reminding myself to switch positions often. Plus, I was not getting the comfort that I needed to handle the intense sensations that, at that point, were occurring each minute. Intuitively, I walked to the bathroom to continue labouring on the toilet. Out of all of the positions I had rehearsed, labouring on the toilet was not in the cards for me – or so I thought. However, I listened to my body and did what felt right (my biggest piece of advice for new parents) and thank God I followed through with it.

I told Brian that I was going to the bathroom, where I proceeded to do a reverse squat on the toilet with a pillow supporting my forehead. In a split second, I heard a plop in the toilet, which signalled to me that my waters must have released. It was time. Immediately after, my body went into the bearing-down phase.

My voice became primal in nature, as I yelled for Brian to signal the midwives. He entered the hallway, while I practically screamed the baby out. Moments later, the midwives came into the restroom holding a flashlight, since they knew I'd requested dim, serene lighting.

Amid the chaos, I lifted my squat to allow the midwives more visibility and opportunity to coach me if necessary. Seconds passed and the midwives saw Kristopher's head! I remember the midwives asking whether I wanted to move from the toilet or deliver there – I shook my head 'no,' but could not vocalize, as my body was already pushing the baby out.

In between my screams, I tried to pause to ensure that I was not manually pushing, but letting my body do the work on its own. On the third scream, Kristopher's full body emerged. He was here!

The midwives caught him, quickly wiped him down, and placed him straight into my hands. Walking slowly out of the bathroom and getting onto the bed, I felt time slow down. The first time I met my baby boy felt like the iconic Simba moment from The Lion King *that we all know and love.*

Exhausted, I lay down and cradled Kristopher. When the umbilical cord stopped pulsating and turned white, the midwife cut it. Moments after, Brian removed his shirt for immediate skin-to-skin contact with his new son.

Brian took over and continued welcoming our baby to the world, as the midwives wanted me to focus on the delivery of my placenta. I was lucky – with a few deep breaths and the application of some light pressure, my placenta was birthed. I decided that I did not want to keep it.

Next, the midwives asked if they could evaluate me for tearing and they explained that minor tears can heal on their own and bigger ones needed stitching. At first, I declined and told them that I preferred to have the tearing (if any) heal on its own. In hindsight, I feel grateful that Brian and the midwives were persistent in suggesting that I get evaluated. Sure enough, I had a second-degree tear and a minor labia tear that needed stitching. If I'm being completely honest, I felt disappointed that I needed stitches. During my pregnancy, I self-administered perineal massages to prevent tearing and I was surely hoping for it to work. The midwives nipped my negative thinking right in the bud by assuring me that I did an incredible job, proclaiming that I must have given birth in a past life! They applauded me on my control throughout the entire process, and that reassurance was all I needed.

While I was getting stitched up, I did not get to breastfeed Kristopher as I had hoped. However, I reminded myself that I could breastfeed my baby when the stitching was over or when we arrived home. By the time they had finished stitching the tears, baby boy was knocked out and our new family of three was ready to head home! Yes, I know what you're thinking. Leaving within a couple of hours of giving birth? That's why I loved using a birthing centre and having a natural delivery!

CHAPTER 9

Preparing for Labour and Birth

We've taken a look at the emotional side of birth, but we all know it's a pretty mammoth physical task too, so in addition to practising your breathing techniques daily, how else can you help your body and mind to prepare for the big day? This chapter will walk you through some key areas to focus on as you prepare for your labour.

Pelvic floor muscles

Your body is magnificent, perfectly designed to create and hold a baby for 40 or so weeks. However, I'm not going to try and kid anyone, growing a human being puts a lot of stress and strain on our body, even when we come from a natural default setting of being fit, strong and healthy. One of the areas that quite literally takes its fair share of the load is the pelvic floor.

Your pelvic floor is made up of the muscles that run from the base of your pubic bone to the back of your spine. Imagine them shaped a little like a hammock or a sling keeping everything else in place. Most of us won't think about stress incontinence in relation to ourselves – even for a moment – until pregnancy kicks in, when people suddenly can't stop going on about how important the pelvic floor is. Looking after your pelvic floor during pregnancy means that you:

- are less likely to leak urine after birth
- are less likely to experience vaginal prolapse (when your pelvic organs begin to bulge into the vagina)
- will boost your post-baby sex life.

— Tip —

If you would like an in-depth look at what you can do to increase and protect your pelvic floor, check out our Pilates Masterclass with Dr Joanna Helcke, at www./thecalm birthschool.com/bookbonuses. However, a great starting point for your pelvic floor preparations are the exercises outlined below.

Pelvic floor techniques

While you may be familiar with the old school squeeze-and-hold exercises, things have moved on considerably since then. Claire Mockridge, a Nutritious Movement™ certified Restorative Exercise Specialist (www.clairemockridge.com) explains below what's changed, and offers the most effective way to prepare your pelvic floor for birth.

Up until a few years ago, pregnant and postnatal women and people were advised to perform traditional pelvic floor exercises known as 'Kegels' to help strengthen the pelvic floor ready for birth. These exercises were invented in the 1940s and involve 'squeezing and releasing' the muscles up to 30 times a day, and 'drawing up and holding', working up to a 10-second hold. However, Kegel exercises are more suitable if you spend most of your day on your feet, whereas many women today have a tight pelvic floor musculature from years of excessive sitting, and doing so in very poor alignment.

Basic anatomy tells us that the pelvic floor muscles run from the pubic bone at the front of your pelvis, to the tailbone at the back. And if you sit with your tailbone tucked underneath you, you're effectively moving the tailbone closer to the pubic bone and passively shortening your pelvic floor. So, learning how to sit correctly for optimum pelvic floor health is a must.

Being in a seated position for work, rest and play takes its toll on the body: your hamstrings, hip flexors and calf muscles all become tighter, and because you're sitting on your gluteal muscles (butt) these aren't getting a workout at all (and neither is your pelvic floor).

Ideally, you'll want all the muscles that feed in and out of the pelvis at their ideal length and strength for the pelvic floor to function well and enable everything to 'give' during childbirth.

Gaining flexibility into the hip flexors and hamstrings with regular stretching exercises and also strengthening the gluteal muscles by performing plenty of squats, lunges and other butt-building, body-conditioning exercises is really a good starting point.

Is it possible to create length in the pelvic floor to enable you to give birth with as little damage as possible? Yes, it is, and the following two exercises will create length in your hamstrings, help you keep your pelvis mobile and ease those aches and pains in your lower back and pelvis.

Hamstring stretch

The hamstrings attach into the back of the pelvis, so lengthening them helps move the tailbone away from the pubic bone, which in turn opens up space for your baby to move through the birth canal.

How to do it

1. Set your feet hip-width apart with your toes pointing forward.

2. Place your hands on a table or on the back of a chair and move your pelvic weight back behind you. Imagine you're reaching your sit bones away from you/relaxing your hip bones down towards the floor.

3. Drop your ribcage down towards your pelvis and stay here for a few minutes. Keep your arms straight and your shoulders relaxed.

When to do it

Do as many reps of this exercise as feels comfortable or for about 10–15 minutes three to five times a week.

Pelvic rocking

Another great movement to strengthen your pelvic floor is one that you can do anywhere when standing, (even in labour) to help keep your pelvis mobile, release tension in your inner thighs and lengthen the pelvic floor muscles.

How to do it

1. Place your feet wider apart with the outside edges of your feet straight.

2. Position your hands on a chair, table or kitchen countertop and, as you tip forward at the hips, reach your sit bones away from you.

3. Keeping your legs straight gently rock your pelvis over to the right, then the left, feeling a lengthening sensation in the inner thighs.

4. Drop your ribcage down towards your pelvis.

When to do it

Do as many reps of this exercise as feels comfortable or for about 10–15 minutes three to five times a week.

Perineal massage

The perineum is the area between the opening of your vagina and your anus. When you're labouring it gets extremely thin as it stretches, so try massaging your perineum to help prevent any damage and reduce the likelihood of tearing or episiotomy – especially if this is a first labour.

Perineal massage technique

This doesn't tend to be a favourite with pregnant people, and I can't understand why! All joking aside, the more familiar you are with your vagina, the more connected you'll feel to yourself and your baby. So don't feel embarrassed. If you find manoeuvring around your curves and bumps a bit awkward, ask your partner to get involved or wait until you're in the bath. However, if you feel totally uncomfortable with the idea of perineum massage, you might like to try an excellent product called EPI-NO. Visit https://epi-no.co.uk/ to find out more about it.

How to do it

Start by washing your hands and then lie down on your side, adding a few drops of a vegetable-based oil, like grapeseed or almond oil, to liberally coat your thumb or index and middle finger.

Insert your fingers into your vagina and gently massage and stretch the area in a U-shape motion.

If you have difficulty reaching the perineum from this angle, standing up and placing a foot on a chair in front of you is a position that many women find provides them with easier access.

When to do it

Start perineal massage from around 36 weeks into your pregnancy and do it for about five minutes once or twice per week.

Prenatal bonding

Prenatal bonding is a hugely important part of the process of becoming a parent. It helps you to tune in to your baby and your body, which is invaluable when you're birthing because it helps you to feel even more of an instant connection with your baby. For partners, it is an excellent way to create a bond with their babies before birth, which not only helps create a sense of involvement for the partner during pregnancy, but also helps them feel more of an immediate bond with baby once they have arrived.

It's not unusual for some partners to take up to six months to bond with their new babies. The time you spend preparing as a couple for your baby's arrival can be hugely beneficial to the attachment process, and prenatal bonding can help to take things to the next level.

Prenatal bonding involves acknowledging and interacting with your baby on a playful and emotional level while they're in the womb. It's easy to recognize our babies are growing physically within us, as our stomachs look fuller every day, but tuning in to how our babies are growing on an emotional level isn't something we always consider.

While we can start prenatal bonding at any time, the last trimester is when our baby's brain development kicks into overdrive. This is the time when our babies are laying down all their instinctive patterns of behaviour as they spend 80 per cent of their time in the REM (rapid eye movement) state. REM is the state of consciousness you enter whenever you're learning something new. Child psychologists talk about what happens between birth and three years of age being crucial, as our children will spend 60 per cent of their time in REM state, downloading much of what is going on around them, creating the templates by which they will live their lives. By the time we are adults we only spend around 20 per cent of time forming these templates, unless we utilize tools like hypnosis, which allow us to enter into this state of conscious, helping us to learn new patterns of behaviour more quickly and easily.

During the last 12 weeks of pregnancy, your baby will learn to look at a human face when they are born. They will learn how to grab hold of your finger instinctively, if you place it in their hand, and they will also know they can mimic and copy, which is why if a person pokes their tongue out at a newborn within the first 24 hours, many babies will return the favour. Being able to mimic, engage and hold on are all vital skills for survival, as they help to promote bonding and attachment with parents immediately post-birth.

Babies communicate with us through their movements, responding to our thoughts, emotions and our external environments, which are all inextricably linked, as far as I'm concerned. Perhaps this is why pregnant women and people often report that a baby who has been relatively quiet throughout the day will start kicking and stretching like crazy whenever they start listening to their audio downloads. I like to think this is baby giving the nod to all the wonderful endorphins coursing around the body.

This is also why some pregnant women and people worry about the impact of stress, anxiety and anger on their babies. While it is true being exposed to consistently stressful situations during your pregnancy isn't ideal, it's not a good idea to beat yourself up every time you experience a cross word with your partner or find yourself in a stressful situation. In fact, a little bit of a difficult episode is the perfect time to practise your

TCBS techniques. Being able to turn instinctively to the breathing exercises that help you return to a feeling of emotional calm when faced with those unavoidable difficult or challenging situations takes practice. So embrace these situations, as it's your ability to tune in to that calming space within that is exactly what you're going to need to do when you're birthing.

You're also teaching your baby the same valuable skill.

While we all instinctively want to protect our children from any difficult emotions or encounters, real life means they will face these situations regularly. It's likely that at some point during your pregnancy you'll feel stressed or frustrated with your partner. This generates stress hormones. However, when you call upon your Calm Birth School tools, your baby gets to experience the return to calm as your body responds with endorphins when you choose to focus on your breath. The lesson you teach your baby here, as they already start to develop their own emotional intelligence, is that even after a storm things always return to a state of calm. The message is that everything will always be all right, which is a very beautiful gift.

So, what can you do to help with this bonding and learning now?

Relax

Every time you access a state of relaxation, listening to your audios and visualizing your baby being born, you're strengthening the bond and connection between the two of you, as well as creating future memories for your hard drive.

Talk and read to your baby

Baby can start hearing your heartbeat and distinguishing between sounds and voices from around 23 weeks. Getting your partner to talk to or read to baby regularly is a great way to start getting familiar with each other.

Massage your bump

Another great way to get your partner involved is gently massaging your bump while talking to you both. Your baby gets to associate your partner with the feel-good hormones, endorphins.

Play games

Responding to your baby's kicks can be both reassuring and a great way to have fun with your baby before they arrive.

Sing

They don't care if you sound like Beyoncé or not, they find dulcet tones reassuring, so sing it out!

Music

Playing the same songs so baby becomes familiar is another great helper and settler once baby arrives: they will associate your favourite pregnancy songs with being safe and secure in the womb.

Understanding estimated due dates

As you start thinking specifically about the big day, it's worth turning your attention to your guess date, or as the professionals like to call it, your estimated due date (EDD). I totally get it – being pregnant for 40 weeks, particularly if you're one of the early birds who knew as soon as you conceived, is a really long time! But eventually, the day arrives: your magic estimated due date.

If you're like the majority of the pregnant population, your ankles have somehow merged with your calves, your rings no longer fit your fingers, you haven't been sleeping well for weeks or months, you're tired of wanting to go to the lavatory every hour, only to realize you can barely squeeze out a wee that would fill a pipette and turning over in the middle of the night feels like trying to shift the Taj Mahal. I remember it well. Your EDD shines down on you like a beacon of hope. Not only is it the day you supposedly get to meet your gorgeous little bundle of joy, but the many, many other benefits that come with giving birth make you cling onto your due date like a limpet on a rock face.

The problem with this though, is that 96 per cent of us are being led up the river without a paddle. For most of us, the day arrives and... nothing: nada, zip, diddly squat. This is for a number of good reasons. The 40-week EDD is based upon Naegele's Rule, a theory developed in 1744 by Harmanni Boerhaave, a botanist. Boerhaave came up with a method of calculating the estimated due date based upon evidence in the Bible indicating human gestation lasts approximately 10 lunar months. The formula was publicized around 1812 by German obstetrician Franz Naegele and since then has become the accepted norm for calculating the due date.

However, there are more than a couple of massive question marks in Naegele's theory.

Strictly speaking, a lunar (or synodic – from new moon to new moon) month is actually 29.53 days, which makes 10 lunar months roughly 295 days, a full 15 days longer than the 280-day gestation we've been led to believe is average. In fact, if left alone, 50–80 per cent of mothers will gestate beyond 40 weeks. I've always gone against conventional wisdom and insisted that pregnancy is a 10-month process.

While your period may have managed to get in sync with a group of friends before, the reality is that we all have different cycles. Even when you know the date of conception, there is a five-week variance with healthy mothers and people giving birth to healthy babies. So, if you give birth at 37 weeks, you're not three weeks early and, if you give birth at 42 weeks, you're not two weeks late. You're only post-date once you exceed 42 weeks.

You might be surprised to learn that only 4 per cent of women give birth on their due date, which is why I prefer to call it a guess date. Remember the power of language (*see page xxv*)? From the moment you're told your guess date, I strongly advise you to do your best to forget it. If you find that the midwives at your antenatal appointments are slightly obsessed with it, don't worry: it's their job to be. Make your peace with knowing it, but perhaps don't share the specifics with your friends and family. The last thing you want is people messaging you and asking, 'Are you still pregnant?' which is beyond annoying. Instead start telling people that you're due around the middle or end of the month (or even two weeks after your guess date, if you want to say a date!), to relieve yourself of any additional pressure. This might feel like you're being dishonest, but it's really an act of self-care, so that as you approach and possibly pass your guess date, you're not being hounded with messages and phone calls checking up on you.

∞ Leanne's birth story ∞

I knew I wanted a home birth. This was my fourth baby and due in the middle of a pandemic, in the second lockdown. I was so organized with this baby, my birth plan was two pages long and really specific to what I wanted, what I needed, what I wanted from my birth team and from Chris, my partner.

I went to my midwife appointment on my EDD and was told I was in slow labour. She didn't monitor me or do an internal – she said she could tell by looking at me. I declined a vaginal examination and a sweep. At 10:30 p.m., I called my midwife and because I was in discomfort and having slight twinges, I asked if she could come and examine me at my house. She said she could do a sweep if I'd like. I accepted a sweep this time. She asked Chris to inflate the pool as I'd definitely be needing it soon. I went to bed and got some sleep.

At 1:20 a.m., I woke up and could not get comfy at all. I was getting twinges in my lower back and the urge to wee! I went to the loo and after timing the surges, I woke Chris up at 2:30 a.m. He rang the midwives and told them I was 'mooing'!

While we were waiting for the midwives, Chris filled the pool and I stood leaning on the back of my nursing chair, rocking from side to side. Chris put Smooth FM on our Alexa, but I couldn't concentrate on my breathing, so Classic FM went on instead so I could stay in my 'zone' – Chris holding my hips from behind and massaging them while I was focusing on my breathing and eating jelly babies!

At 3 a.m., I decided to get into the pool and get myself into a comfortable position. I was leaning over the side, tummy fully submerged in the water, and I was so relaxed, the atmosphere was calm and chilled. While waiting for the midwives, me and Chris enjoyed a lovely cup of tea together while I was in the pool.

The midwives arrived at 3:15 a.m. – all three of them! The first midwife came and sat by me and asked how I was feeling and if I needed anything, I said I was fine, and that I didn't need anything. Chris gave each of them my birth plan while they set up a little area for themselves and for the baby. At 4:20 a.m. we were joined by an unexpected guest: my daughter Eden had woken up and come down the stairs. It was a really hot summer, so seeing me in the pool wasn't an unusual sight – she didn't bat an eyelid! She loved that there were new people to show her toys to and she and a midwife became great friends! I loved concentrating on watching her play and maybe having Eden present was the boost of oxytocin I wanted and needed. But at 4:45, I gave Chris the thumbs up and said I was ready to guide our baby. I had a midwife holding my hand and guiding my breaths, Chris telling me how much he loved me and that I could do this, another midwife playing with Eden and another one sat observing from the other side of the pool.

I remember asking if I was crowning – the midwife said I had pooed! I was actually relieved as I had been constipated for three days! She then informed me my waters had released and asked if I was ready to catch my little boy. I put my hands down between my legs and caught him after one down-breath at 4:58 a.m. I held him in the water while I turned round to bring him up to my chest.

I took in the environment: Chris watching me, the midwives observing me, Eden playing – and I was sitting in the pool holding my baby. It was all calm and still; no one was in any rush to check me or Jacob. It was silent while I brought him out of the water and held him against me as he let out his first breath and his cry, bringing Eden running over to meet her baby brother!

Chris handed me a towel for him and for my shoulders. I held the cord in my hand for delayed cord clamping and notified the midwives when it had stopped pulsing and was white. Chris cut the cord, with Eden supervising as she was in awe of her baby brother. The midwives passed Jacob to Chris to help me out of the pool to birth my placenta earthside as I'd wanted to have it encapsulated.[44] The midwives filled out the paperwork for this.

The midwife wrapped me in a big fluffy dressing gown and helped me onto the sofa before checking me down there for grazes or tears; all was fine so she handed Jacob back to me, Chris and Eden joined me while the midwives tidied up and made us all tea and toast in my home! Jacob was weighed at 6:45 a.m., weighing 9lb 6oz, to the amazement of all of us!

At 7:30 a.m., the midwives had gone home to get some well-earned rest and we were left in our cosy bubble of love and comfort.

CHAPTER 10

Your Birth Partner's Role

When Suzy used to teach hypnobirthing to couples face to face, she would always joke that the birth partner was supposed to be a bit like Batman: the one with all the tools, techniques and knowledge about how to support you best on the day you meet your baby. Many of the pregnant women and people who take The Calm Birth School video course or classes hosted by a TCBS Instructor love the fact that their partners can get a full picture of what they can do by learning exactly what they, as birthing people, are learning.

The role of the birth partner begins long before labour. If you haven't been sharing the tools and the philosophy of the book, make sure that you start sharing them now. Your birth partner's energy on the day you go into labour will have a profound impact on how you're feeling, even if this is at a subconscious level.

This information applies to male birth partners, same-sex couples, mothers, sisters, friends, birthing partners who don't identify as male, non-binary individuals and trans birth partners too – basically anyone who is going to be your primary support.

It's quite easy when we look at the stereotypes of birth to feel that it is a one-woman or -person show. How we feel in the lead-up to our baby's birth day and how we feel on the day is very much a team effort. So, to reiterate, make sure your partner reads this chapter if nothing else. This is especially for them.

During pregnancy

The gift of listening is one of the biggest gifts your birth partner can give you. Being heard during your pregnancy and birth is one of the biggest dictators of how a birthing woman or person perceives their experience. And while it's very easy at times to think your partner knows, or should already know, what you want, often they don't. This isn't their fault; it is just one of those things. So, getting in some dedicated listening time is a priority. The by-product of this will be confidence that your birth partner knows what you want and will be capable of working with your care providers to help you stay calm and positive throughout. And perhaps, most importantly, it will foster a deeper connection between the two of you.

If you already feel you have a great foundation for listening, use the next exercise to build on what you have already, and if you know that you and your birth partner could use a little help with getting on the same page when it comes to your wants and desires for your birth, then this is the perfect opportunity to create the space to connect.

Listening with intention

The great news about this technique, as with all the techniques in the book, is that it isn't rocket science, but it will take a little effort from both of you to make it happen.

How to do it

Take some time out together. We've talked about the importance of taking some dedicated time for yourself every day (*see Chapter 2, page 14*), but spending time with your partner talking about the birth is magical. And while the emphasis in the earlier weeks is likely to be on birth choices, how you're feeling and any worries or concerns, this is also a fantastic forum for both of you to discuss your expectations, plans, ideas and again, any worries or concerns you may have about being a parent for the first time, or again.

How to do it

The only rules are: no technology, and when one of you is talking, the other person has to listen.

Here are my top tips for listening with intention:

* **Don't interrupt:** Don't look for the next opportunity to say what you think, even if you agree with what your birth partner is saying – be present.

* **Make eye contact:** Reflect back what your partner is saying to you before you add your personal comments to make sure you have heard and understood what has been said.

When to do it

Aim to sit down together at least once a week, and if your birth partner is away during your pregnancy, then downtime together can be just as effectively achieved over Skype, Zoom or FaceTime. If you're unable to have any contact with your birth partner during your pregnancy, do not stress out about it. Just make sure you prime them once they return, so that they can support you by reading this chapter of the book. It's also a good idea to write a list of any questions, concerns or things that are important to you, or you would like them to consider so you can discuss them once you get the opportunity.

. . . .

Learn the breathing techniques

I can't emphasize enough how useful it is for your birth partner to learn the breathing techniques with you (*see The Calm Birth School Breathing Techniques at a Glance, page 259*). Your birth partner will know you better than anyone in the room, after all the quality downtime you have been spending together, and is the person to whom you're likely to have the strongest emotional bond.

There is no doubt you'll pick up on the energy they are emitting while you're labouring and birthing. If they are anxious, worried or concerned about you or the process, they will be producing their own adrenaline and cortisol, so they will then have to focus on managing the fight–flight–freeze response (*see Chapter 1, page 9*) rather than focusing on you and your needs, or are unable to respond or manage what is going on outside of themselves as effectively.

The biggest problem with your birth partner feeling stressed is the potential for you to pick up on those emotions. It's a bit like walking into a room where a couple have been arguing and you can feel the tension and negative energy lingering even though nothing is being said. If you notice that your partner is feeling stressed, either consciously or subconsciously, the impact can cause you to lose focus or, on a subconscious level, fear there is something to worry about. So having a birth partner who can manage their own range of emotions is paramount. And, as you already know, one of the best tools for helping you to regain a sense of peace, calm and control is to regulate the breath.

If your partner is instinctively taking long, slow, deep breaths because of all the practice they have done and radiating a sense of calm and peace, you're far more likely to pick up on it and adjust your breathing accordingly, without them needing to tell you to do anything differently. This means they can guide you into relaxing and lengthening your breath without any need for a conversation.

It can also help to avoid unwittingly pushing your buttons by saying things like, 'remember to breathe', or 'are you doing TCBS breathing now?' They just take the lead and set the example to you by demonstrating long, deep, audible breaths.

Massage

We'll look at the power of positive touch in a later chapter because, although you may not want this type of touch during labour, if you become accustomed to being massaged by your partner during pregnancy, the positive associations will help you in labour – even if all you do is hold hands. If you get used to visualizing birthing your baby while your partner is touching you during pregnancy, then you strengthen the association between you and your partner when it comes to your baby's birth. At least 10 minutes a day of light touch massage is just what the TCBS orders.

Bag packing

Write out a checklist of all the items you think you might need during your labour. This is a really positive thing to do, even if you're birthing at home, for the following reasons:

- You'll have everything you need all in one place.

- If you change your mind and decide you would prefer to birth in hospital, or special circumstances arise that make sense for you to move locations, your birth partner won't miss anything vital off the list.

> **— Tip —**
>
> Get your birth partner to pack the bag for you. This isn't being lazy, but will help your birth partner to know exactly what's in the bag and where to find anything you might need. It's also useful to keep the checklist on top of the bag, so should you ask for anything, your partner can quickly scan the list to check that it's in there, without needing to ask you.

On the day

Throughout labour and delivery, remember that your birth partner is your servant. No joke. Your birth partner is responsible for ensuring that you're super comfortable in early labour and that you have everything you need.

Early labour

The early phase of labour – particularly if your birth partner will be co-parenting with you – can be a fantastic time for bonding and connecting before your baby arrives. So what can you do with your partner to make this moment, a moment?

Use these moments to tune in to each other – and the fact that life will never be quite the same again – in the best possible way. This part of your labour can be deeply, deeply romantic and intimate, especially first time around.

Your excitement should be palpable, and you can, if you want, turn this part of your pregnancy and birth into a beautiful moment. You might choose to go for a walk together, light some candles, listen to music, enjoy a massage, look into each other's eyes and celebrate what's happening. If that sounds a bit too soppy for you – don't worry: find your own way to take stock and connect. However, this bonding is important because the more you can feel as though you, your baby and your partner are working together, the more oxytocin you can't help but produce, which often means an easier labour. Your birth partner can play a vital role in helping you to generate oxytocin. This may be by making you laugh, offering reassuring pep talks, kissing, hugging, massage, slow dancing, nipple stimulation, or any or all the above that will raise your mood. If you decide you would prefer to take this time for yourself, of course, that is OK too, just focus on spending time on activities that make you smile and increase your endorphin and oxytocin levels.

If this is baby number two or more, it can definitely be more challenging to create the type of intimacy I have outlined above, but don't be defeated. If your older child or children are present, consider what you can do to make this a family moment instead? Perhaps it's still going for a walk in the park, letting them know that the baby brother or sister will be here sooner rather than later. Or maybe ask a friend or family member to babysit, so you don't need to focus on keeping them entertained. There is no right or wrong answer to what to do with older children during labour and birth. Just do what makes sense for you and the family.

While not quite as romantic, other practical things your partner can do are to remind you to use your birth ball, make sure your musical playlist is ready and that you have funny films on tap. Have all of your liquids and snacks ready and know where the birth bag is, of course.

> ## — Tip —
>
> Be mindful of not going into deep relaxation mode straight away – it's totally fine for you to keep active for as long as feels comfortable for you. Just make sure you have enough snacks, drinks, your birth playlist and audio downloads to hand, and that you are comfortable.

At the hospital

Once you're at the hospital, your birth partner can make sure your care providers have a copy of your birth preferences and have read through them and know where the spare copy has been tucked away too.

While you settle in, your birth partner can get busy making sure that the birth suite is as comfortable as possible, and that everyone in the room is in tune with your wishes. And should they notice someone that isn't on the same page as you, ensuring they speak to the consultant midwife or whoever is in charge to see if they can allocate another member of staff to your team.

Other practical considerations might include:

- lowering the lighting or putting up LED candles around the room
- placing pictures in optimal positions
- setting up your device so you can listen to your music or TCBS audio downloads
- breathing with you slowly and audibly.

For the most part, your birth partner will play the role of the silent observer, unless you're up for having a chat in between your surges, of course. They will also:

- be on the lookout for any build-up of tension in your face or body and assisting you by remembering to breathe themselves
- be ready to hold you or touch you, as hand holding or light touch massage can be great to help support you during a surge, if you're open to it (*see also page 131*)
- whisper words of encouragement
- encourage you to drink fluids regularly and eat to keep your strength up
- remind you to go to the lavatory every 45 minutes or so, as babies do not like passing full bladders
- and, most importantly, they remember to be present.

❧ A birth partner's story ❧

Alex and I went for an early walk at about 8:30 a.m. around the village. We came back early as Alex needed to wee. As she went to the toilet, her plug fell out and we knew the birth could be round the corner. I had to leave for work at 11:30 a.m. and I was working until 9 p.m. I made sure my phone was on loud ALL day! On coming home, Alex was fine, but her stomach was tingling, and Braxton Hicks surges were getting stronger. We slept OK that evening.

I was really hesitant to go to work the next day. I just didn't want to be away from Alex at all. There was an enormous amount of guilt as I left for work. At 6 p.m. I got home, and Alex thought she needed yet another wee. It turned out it was actually her waters trickling down her leg. She called the hospital and told them what had happened, and they asked her to come in with an overnight bag. Our hearts were racing as it was now... it was really happening!

Alex had a shower and shouted from the stairs... 'OMG, my waters have properly broken.' It was all over the carpet!

We got to the hospital and the staff were lovely. They examined Alex but couldn't see how many centimetres she was dilated. At 9 p.m. they sent us back home, as we weren't in established labour.

At home, neither of us slept. Alex's surges were getting stronger and then she had a bloody show. We called the hospital again and they told us to come straight in. Little did we know, that was the last time we were leaving the house as a couple.

At the hospital once more, Alex was assessed. She was 5cm and we both smiled at one another.

We showed our birth notes to our midwife and explained we were Hypnobirthing. We also explained we would like a water birth. This had been in question previously, due to Alex having low iron levels. Thankfully, her iron levels were now good enough. They said there was one birth pool left, which was amazing to hear.

We went into the pool room, put some music on and I created that birth environment. Alex got used to how the gas and air worked, and they started to fill the pool up. This was at around 12:30 a.m. We knew we had missed our due date and we were now into Thursday.

Her next assessment was at 4:30 a.m. and the surges were getting stronger. She was now 7cm.

The next steps were the hardest. I've never seen a stronger woman in my life, and I couldn't be more proud of her. Alex used gas and air the whole time, kneeling over the pool with her hands in mine. Using the breathing techniques we learned in our Hypnobirthing classes with Leanne, I gently coached her through.

I felt as though I played a huge part in her pain relief. I kept asking her to look me in the eye and I was just smiling back. There were moments when I was running to and from the sink rinsing a cold towel to put around her shoulders.

She was now in serious labour and everything is a slight blur from then onwards... however there are some important moments I recall. The next examination for Alex was due at 8:30 a.m., but they got her out of the birth pool early – our midwife could tell the baby was near. I asked the midwife to tell me how dilated Alex was, as I did not want her to be disappointed. She was fully dilated. I told Alex this and kissed her on the forehead. She knew she was near... from then, it happened so quickly.

The midwife told Alex to let her body now do the work, and this is where her breathing changed. I suggested, 'Let's change it to breathe out from the nose.' By this time, anything goes – so most of her breathing was done through her mouth. She was making some noises I never knew existed... ha ha!

Alex did not manage to get back in the birth pool after her examination. She started to give birth on the cushion bed next to the birthing pool. The midwife said she could feel the head was near and it started coming.

Now here is when panic set in. Our midwife, Tracey, was amazing. We were told she needed a second opinion on something, so she asked for some help. Help – the whole bloody hospital and their dogs arrived! Nine ladies entered the room and I'll be honest, we shat ourselves. Indie's heart rate dropped quite a lot but came back up.

The second time, it stayed low, so they had to act quickly. I tried to keep Alex calm still, as she was pretty out of it. I was amazed at how professional and how quickly the hospital staff made critical decisions.

They asked Alex to get up off the cushion bed, but she couldn't. A wheelchair was sourced for her, and with a little assistance Alex was whisked down the corridor mid-contraction, with no pain relief. They took us from the midwife-led unit to the delivery ward.

Alex was helped onto a proper bed, legs in stirrups. We were told our baby's shoulders were slightly twisted, so she didn't have enough room to descend. This was causing baby to panic. A midwife made a small cut to give our baby some more space. Another midwife then asked Alex to breathe in, chin on chest, and pretend she was having a big poo. I reminded Alex, 'Breathe out through your nose.'

One... two... three massive pushes and she was out. We were parents. Our daughter was born at 9:49 a.m. and weighed 7lb 7oz. Due date plus 1.

I was so proud of Alex and our daughter Indie. It must have been hard for her inside, trying to come out too.

After our birth, Alex decided to stay in overnight. She didn't feel comfortable coming home after all the exhaustion. I came home, but could not sleep or eat, I was just thinking of them both constantly.

At 9 a.m. on the Friday, following a few successful breastfeeds, we headed home. I drove at 5mph all the way home.

CHAPTER 11

Induction and
Special Circumstances

Remember, the thing that gets your labour going is oxytocin – the hormone of 'luurve' (*see Chapter 3, page 36*). If your guess date has been and gone and you're getting tense and frustrated because your baby doesn't seem ready to make an appearance, remember your estimated due date is a guess date (*see Chapter 9, page 121*). Then have a word with yourself and partake in some oxytocin-inducing, relaxation-friendly activities.

However, sometimes for reasons and situations beyond our control, special circumstances arise sometime before our guess dates or we require assistance from our care providers during labour. It is in these special circumstances that all of your training in staying calm, using your BRAIN and really leaning into the idea that you can still enjoy a positive birth experience, even if you're not getting your Plan A preferences, comes into play. And when it comes to hearing the many different birth stories, it's often these stories that have the biggest impact on us, as birthing women and people describe how they were able to navigate the twists and turns of labour from a position of strength and control.

Continuous monitoring

Depending on the nature of your pregnancy you might find yourself in a position where you're invited to have continuous monitoring before or during your birth. This situation may occur if:

- you have high blood pressure
- you have or develop pregnancy-related diabetes
- your waters have released and more than 24 hours have passed
- you have had a caesarean birth in the past
- your waters have released and there is meconium (baby poo) in the water and the baby doesn't appear to be stressed
- you're expecting twins.

It is incredibly important that you use the BRAIN system (*see Chapter 7, page 74*), and ask your care providers about the risks and benefits of being continuously monitored in your specific situation, and particularly if the reasons are non-medical – such as having had a previous caesarean birth or you're expecting twins, for example. You do have options. The research shows that, while continuous foetal monitoring reduces the chances of neonatal seizure in-utero, it also increases the chances of having a caesarean birth or assisted delivery.[45] So please do your homework. You always have a choice.

Pre-labour interventions

The reason that so many people spend time discussing the arbitrary 40-week EDD is because this date plays a big role in determining whether a pregnant woman or person will be advised or offered a pre-labour intervention, and if you're hoping for an intervention-free birth this is a big deal. However, when it comes to pre-labour interventions, I want you to put the 'shoulds' out with the rubbish.

If there is no medical reason for you to need intervention – i.e. you're experiencing a low-risk pregnancy but reach 41+3 weeks and decide you just have to meet this baby and would like some assistance from your medical team to help this process along, then this is your right to choose to do so too – just as it is your right to refuse it.

Sometimes, what you want will be moral support to remind you that you really are on the home straight and will be meeting your baby soon enough. At other times, you'll just want to get on with it. And it's during those times you may be presented with the following options:

Stretch and sweep

Depending on the local policy of your care providers, once a pregnant woman or person passes their EDD they may be offered a stretch and sweep. This is where your care provider will use their fingers to massage the neck of the cervix, in the hope of stimulating the uterus and kick-starting labour.

Although to be offered a sweep is common, studies have shown varying results. Some research indicates that it is effective, while others have shown that there is no difference in waiting. Although evidence may indicate that it does have its advantages, the disadvantages need to be addressed also.[46] For instance, it doesn't always work, and the procedure can be uncomfortable, causing both bleeding and cramping. It could encourage stop/start surges, which can be exhausting, and there is a possibility of the procedure prematurely releasing your waters.[47] As with all interventions, a stretch and sweep can only be carried out with informed consent, so you'll need to make up your mind as to whether you feel happy with moving forward with a sweep or not. Depending on where you're based, this intervention can be offered prior to 40 weeks. Some may decide that they do not want any form of intervention at all; others feel that when faced with a possible chemical induction they would rather give the 'less invasive' option a try. Neither decision is right or wrong. This is your body, your birth and your baby. You have to do what feels right for you.

Induction

If you're experiencing a low-risk pregnancy, it is unusual to be offered an induction prior to your EDD. However, an increase in blood pressure, a prolonged start to labour after waters releasing, or concern over baby's growth rate, are all reasons that it may be recommended.

While hospital policy will vary from region to region, once a pregnant woman or person reaches 41+1 weeks, and particularly if they are birthing in a hospital, their caregiver is likely to start discussing the option of booking in an induction.

Inductions are an extremely emotive subject within the birth world. Many birth professionals would advise that women and birthing people should absolutely not be induced unless there are specific medical reasons.

Although we feel alarmed by the rising rate of inductions our view is not so black and white, and this is simply because we don't think being petrified of induction is helpful. We have received many letters from The Calm Birth School students who have used TCBM and experienced incredibly positive births, because they were able to stay calm and in control throughout. In fact, a TCBS Instructor, Jade Gordon, has an entire online course dedicated to creating a positive induction experience and a host of stories that reflect that it is possible.[48]

Having said that, choosing to be induced is a big decision, as a medically managed birth means that your body doesn't produce its own oxytocin and endorphins in the same way as a birth that is able to progress naturally. The consequence of this is that many of the benefits we talk about in terms of being able to enjoy a comfortable and more relaxed birth are more difficult to experience. Often the process makes birth much more intense. However, anecdotally, hypnobirthers who have trained themselves to relax deeply on demand and are able to go with the sensations they experience, as opposed to fighting against their body, are in the best position to still create a more positive induction experience. Go back to being clear on the risks and benefits of moving forward with any procedure during pregnancy and birth and make your decisions based on what feels right for you and your family.

If you do decide to move forward with an induction, my key piece of advice is to build up your bank of endorphins and get your natural oxytocin level as high as possible before going to the hospital. Put the following three priorities at the top of your induction checklist:

1. **Feel happy:** Once you know you're going to be induced, you also know that within a couple of days maximum

you're going to be holding your baby in your arms for the very first time. Woohoo!

2. **Listen to the 'Fear Release' audio download (www. thecalmbirthschool.com/shop/):** Acknowledge any fears or anxiety about being induced you might be holding on to and then let them go.

3. **Make more endorphins:** Start building up your bank of endorphins by spending time with your partner and in activities that make you feel happy and relaxed, whether that's making love or cuddling your partner, watching funny movies, drawing.

— Tip —

If you're in need of inspiration, check out the suggestions for creating more oxytocin in Chapter 10 (*see page 133*) or listen to the Calm Birth Hypnobirthing Meditation via the *Empower You: Unlimited Audio* mobile app.

Building up your bank of natural endorphins so you feel more relaxed and at ease before your induction will help you manage the stronger surges more effectively so you can work with your body as opposed to against it. And should you start surging regularly, you can always request that you continue to labour without further stimulation. (I recommend putting this in your birth preferences.)

And to reiterate: you'll still be able to use the techniques outlined in this book should you go in for an induction. In fact, it's very important that you do and because you'll know your date for induction, you'll have a head start! So use this to your advantage.

The induction process

Most pregnant women and people will have been offered up to two cervical sweeps prior to a medically managed labour. Often, a gel or a pessary containing artificial prostaglandins to help to ripen the cervix and stimulate uterine waves is inserted into the vagina. If this is unsuccessful, you'll be asked if you're open to having your waters artificially released. This is usually done with a small hook that looks similar to a crochet hook. The impact of artificially rupturing your membrane can, in some cases, mean your labour progresses very quickly and intensely. If this isn't enough to get things moving, you'll be offered Syntocinon or Pitocin depending on where you are in the world, which is a synthetic form of oxytocin, administered via intravenous drip.

It is widely thought that the pressure waves stimulated by these artificial drugs ARE much more intense that the body's own natural waves. When induced, the body does not respond by producing endorphins in the same way as when someone goes into labour naturally, which is why your own preparation, should you be having an induction, is so crucial. Everything you have learned and all your practice becomes even more important. If you do have a medically managed birth you'll be offered an epidural to eliminate the pain. This is something some will choose to move forward with immediately, and others choose to wait it out. There is no right or wrong answer to this; only you can decide what is right or wrong for you and your family on the day.

If you decide induction isn't for you, this too is a valid choice, as you do not have to move forward with any medical care, including being induced. This can often feel like a difficult decision to make, which can leave you feeling very isolated unless you're under the care of an independent or private midwife, because you'll be going against the status quo, and your care providers may be against waiting for nature to take its course.

Often pregnant women and people are told they run the risk of their bodies not functioning as effectively if they allow their birth to continue past the 42-week period, alongside risking the health of their babies.

This is something no pregnant person wants to hear, and many tend to proceed with the intervention, despite feeling uncomfortable with the choice, or as if they do not have alternative options. However, the risks, when stated in this fashion, do not present a full picture, which means you're unable to make an informed decision. I strongly recommend that if you're thinking about induction and are not sure whether it is right, you visit www.aims.org.uk (Association for Improvements in the Maternity Services). This charity provides robust statistical, evidence-based research that is extremely accessible for those of us without medical backgrounds. This will allow you to assess whether induction is the right decision for you or not.

Hypnobirthing is about understanding what you can control and letting go of what you can't. In terms of medical interventions, you're always the person in charge. No one can 'not allow' you to do something; you always have the right to make a decision based on informed consent. You have the right to choose not to move forward with an induction. You have the right to decline vaginal examinations. You can choose to birth at home after a previous caesarean. You have the right to ask for evidence to support the advice you're given, and there are many sources of information that you can seek out independently to help you to make an informed choice about how you would like to proceed with your pregnancy and your birth.

> **— Tip —**
>
> When faced with any non-urgent medical matters, use your BRAIN system (Benefits, Risks, Alternatives, Instincts, Nothing – *see Chapter 7, page 74*). Ask questions and do the research so you can look back and know you had the best birth experience for you on the day.

If you decide an induction isn't for you, but you would like to feel even more at ease with your decision, you can request additional monitoring of both you and your baby. You can also ask for the amount of fluid around your baby to be checked, as well as baby's positioning.

Bear in mind that we were not designed to stay pregnant. And barring special circumstances, our body gets it spot on. So if you're experiencing a low-risk pregnancy and all the signs point to a healthy baby, many people would argue your baby hasn't been born yet because your baby is simply not ready. Your body will kick into action when your baby is ready.

Special circumstances

We have already discussed birth preferences and their importance, particularly in situations when birth does not go to plan (see Chapter 7, page 75). While it is extremely important to focus on creating the calm, positive birth you desire, sometimes even with the best planning in the world, special circumstances may mean you'll have to look at your B and C options for birth preferences.

Sometimes, those who end up having pain relief for the intensity of their surges or perhaps meeting an unplanned scenario feel like there has been some kind of failure on their or their body's part. I want to emphasize that no one can fail at birth and your aim is to enjoy an experience that you want to look back on with joy in your heart, whether your baby arrives vaginally, breech, with the help of forceps, an epidural or via caesarean.

All these experiences can be as magical as the next when you feel clear on why certain precautions or actions are taking place, and when it feels right for the health of you and your baby. The aim is always for a positive birth, not a perfect one.

Alongside birth not playing out exactly as we anticipated, for what can be a multitude of non-medical reasons, it's also important for you to be mindful of the clear medical reasons why you should seek out support during your pregnancy or labour should you notice any of the following:

- Feeling your surges start prior to 37 weeks. Although it's very common to experience Braxton Hicks, a tightening of your tummy without much intensity in the latter stages of pregnancy, if you're surging and noticing intensity before the 37-week period you should call your care team straight away.

- If you notice a change in your baby's regular patterns of movement after 24 weeks.[49] Many people mistakenly believe that baby's movement will slow down towards the end of your pregnancy but this isn't the case. Take a look at www.kickscount.org.uk for more information on how to monitor your baby's movements.

- A prolonged period of time from your waters releasing to the onset of labour. We include this tentatively and urge you to do your own research around this, as many are offered antibiotics or inductions on the basis of safety for both birthing person and child when in fact, the evidence to support the normal course of action for most medical care providers suggests that waiting to see if labour progresses normally without any intervention actually poses significantly less risk than what is often presented.[50]

- Noticing that your membranes are discoloured or have a strong odour once your waters have released. This could be meconium (baby's poo), which can be a sign of some distress for baby, while an odour might indicate a urinary tract infection.

- Regular and severe headaches.

- A very high temperature or fever.

- Extreme vomiting or diarrhoea.

- Blurred vision or dizziness, particularly if combined with substantial swelling of hands, face, ankles or feet.

- Heavy bleeding. While it's normal to experience spotting towards the end of term, your care team should immediately check out any heavy bleeding.

As always, don't forget to tune in to and trust your instinct; if something doesn't feel right, even if you can't put your finger on it, receiving reassurance from your care team that everything looks OK and there's nothing to be concerned about is a great endorphin producer, which will always be a good thing for both you and your baby.

Helping birth along naturally

When your baby is almost ready to make an appearance, sometimes it is possible to give them a little encouragement and help them on their way. While I don't believe any of these suggestions will help if your baby's not ready to make an appearance, they can be useful if all baby needs is a little nudge in the right direction to make their appearance. Or if you feel like you 'need' to do something, anything, to encourage this baby out of it's incubation period... of course, you don't need to do anything at all because nature's got you covered, right? But trust me, I know that feeling of just 'wanting to get the baby out'! So here are a few things for you to consider trying out.

Sex

Sex and/or physical intimacy is arguably one of the best things you can do to nudge things along. When we get intimate, particularly when we are climaxing, we produce huge amounts of oxytocin. So touching, kissing and making love are all fantastic ways to encourage labour to start. Prostaglandins, also found in semen, help to soften and ripen the cervix, which in theory can help with dilation.

Reflexology

Reflexology is great at around 36/37 weeks, as a reflexologist skilled in maternity reflexology will stimulate certain pressure points within the body that are known to stimulate labour. Rather than waiting until the final minute as a last resort, think about a course of sessions around the 36-week mark, which are anecdotally reported to be more effective in encouraging babies to arrive closer to their guess date.

Acupuncture

A series of sessions from around 36–37 weeks can be very helpful. Some practitioners offer specific packages for avoiding induction too. Acupuncture originates from Chinese medicine and the methods used work with the body's energy systems and meridians, moving a woman's energy to help baby make an appearance.

Acupressure

This works in a similar way to acupuncture, but without the needles, and focuses on stimulating labour by applying pressure to points across the body.

Being physically active

Walking up stairs and steep hills is great, because you tend to be in a forward-leaning position, which helps get your baby to put more pressure on the cervix in order to help stimulate the uterus into action.

Dates

Eating six dates a day from 36 weeks onwards has been shown to increase the likelihood of spontaneous labour and reduce the chances of intervention.[51]

Nipple stimulation

Using either your hands or a breast pump will help produce the hormone oxytocin, which you'll definitely know by this point is great for stimulating birth.

Spicy food

Any spicy food that might make you want to go to toilet, basically. Kick it up a notch. So, if you're used to eating a madras curry you need to go for a vindaloo or a phal, whereas if you normally love a korma then a madras would be fine.

(... Oh, and did I mention sex?!)

❧ Natalie's birth story ❧

I started having increased baby movements on Tuesday 29 June. He was kicking me so low down that it was painful and uncomfortable. I called the triage for advice and they said this was normal for 28 weeks. It continued into Wednesday so I called them again as I was concerned something was wrong. I was assured it was not. On Wednesday night I started having mild cramps in my tummy. They were like mild period pains and continued through the night on Wednesday.

On Thursday I had a midwife appointment and they believed I was experiencing Braxton Hicks, but the intensity during Thursday night got worse. The cramp-style sensations had increased and they were about every 10 minutes or so. This is when I started using my breathing techniques as learned with The Calm Birth School video course. I lay in my bed and thought, what a good opportunity to practise for the birth. Breathe through and stay calm.

I called the triage again on Friday morning and they were not concerned as the baby was kicking and believed I had an irritated uterus. Friday was a long day. My baby was kicking but the cramps were far less until about 7 p.m. when they started to increase again. I didn't get much sleep that night, I used my breathing during the sensations, which helped but I was uncomfortable. I went to the toilet and noticed blood about 6 a.m. We called triage again and they sent us in to be checked.

I was hooked up to machines for about an hour. They were convinced I had an infection and did not suspect labour. However, when the consultant examined me, I was 5cm dilated. Everything changed – the whole dynamic of the room. Loads of people were around me telling me the baby was coming and they couldn't stop it. They tried to slow him down so they could give me some drugs to help him, but he wasn't having any of it. At the next examination I was 7cm dilated and they could feel his little hand. Emergency C-Section was needed to get him out safely. Everything seemed to speed up: my clothes were being changed, everyone was rushing around. Nurses were telling me what was going on, but in my mind I just knew my only job now was to stay calm and breathe. My baby needed me strong now more than ever, and I was determined that the one thing I was able to do in this situation would be done the best I could. My husband couldn't believe how calm I stayed, regardless of how scared I was.

My son Tyce was born, weighing 2lb 12oz at 28 weeks' gestation. One thing I know for sure is that my birthing experience would have been 10 times worse if it wasn't for The Calm Birth School. This was not the birth I ever anticipated or wanted, but they prepared me for that. Not just for the birth but for all the scary times I have been facing since and will continue to face while Tyce is so young. For that I can't thank The Calm Birth School enough for the education and support I received through my pregnancy.

Caesarean Birth

One of the biggest misconceptions we wanted to bust through our work at The Calm Birth School and using TCBM techniques is the idea that birthing women and people who end up having a caesarean birth, either unplanned or elective, have in some way been let down by their bodies. And in the case of unplanned caesareans have been let down by hypnobirthing or if opting for an elective caesarean, don't think they will benefit from hypnobirthing. We are both here to say that all of that is rubbish.

Unplanned caesarean birth

Historically, unplanned caesareans are often referred to as emergencies. However, emergency isn't always the most accurate way to describe events and by the nature of the emotions generally attached the word emergency isn't the most useful way to describe the procedure, which is why we like to opt for unplanned.

The great thing about unplanned caesarean births when you're using The Calm Birth Method is that you can plan for them beforehand.

Again, while it isn't useful to focus lots of attention on plans B and C, doing so now, getting clear on what you want and what you don't want will serve you well should anything unexpected happen.

So why might your care providers suggest that a caesarean may be the best course of action for you and your baby?

- prolonged first or second stage of labour
- if baby appears to be in any distress
- if baby has manoeuvred into a non-optimal position that will make it difficult for you to labour optimally
- if there is any excessive bleeding.

With most unplanned caesareans, the decision to move forward isn't an urgent one and you'll have time to talk and think it through. This is the time to use your BRAIN (see Chapter 7, page 74). If the situation is urgent, your care team will want and need you to act quickly. This can lead to there being lots of people in the room and lots of hustle and bustle. This is where your breathing techniques really come into play. While you may not be able to control what is going on around you, if you have been practising your breathing techniques in real-life situations, you'll be able to tap in to narrowing your focus of attention so that you keep your breathing slow and long, feeding your uterus and baby with oxygen.

Elective caesarean

If you're opting to have a caesarean for whatever reason again the work that you do during your pregnancy will provide you and your partner with a fantastic foundation for:

- Releasing any fears you may have about going into hospital or having the caesarean birth.

- Helping you and your partner to take time out to bond actively and consciously with baby and the new roles you'll be taking on.

- Providing you with breathing techniques to help both of you stay calm and relaxed during the caesarean birth.

- The breathing and visualization techniques you practise during your pregnancy will also help you to manage any pain you may experience during your recovery too.

Natural caesareans

It's very useful to outline how you would like to experience your caesarean birth in your birth preferences too. Things you might want to consider:

- If having an elective caesarean, ask to see what the operating theatre looks like so you know where you'll be having baby.

- Ask whether you can play your own music.

- Ask whether you can wear your own clothing.

- Request that your hands be kept free from any monitors.

- Any anaesthetic used should not affect the upper part of the body so you can hold your baby as soon as they have been delivered.

- Any intravenous drips are placed in your non-dominant arm.

- Have a think about if you would like the screen lowered. Many women and birthing people like to have it up for the incision and then taken down so they can see their baby being lifted out.

- Where do you want your birth partner to be standing – close to your upper body or closer to baby?

- Do you want immediate skin to skin or would you prefer for baby to cleaned up first?

- How long would you like the umbilical cord to be left for? Although you'll have mentioned this in your ideal birth scenario, it is important to highlight it in the section too if you would like it to go white or at least stop pulsating naturally.

- Would you like you or your partner to cut the umbilical cord?

Having this incredibly gentle start to life, where you dictate how you would like things to happen, can be as powerful and soul-affirming as a vaginal birth, but you have to think about what you want and ensure that your birth partner or you are able to communicate those wants effectively. Caesarean mothers and people give birth too, and we want you to own it.

CHAPTER 13

Signs of Early Labour

Early labour is known as the 'latent phase'. Contrary to popular belief, not all of us will 'just know' when we have gone into labour. Some of us will, but if you find yourself second-guessing all the usual aches and twinges as you approach or pass your guess date, do not fear. You're not alone. To help determine if this really is your moment, here are seven helpful hints of what to look out for.

The seven signs of early labour

1. Excessive nesting

Most people will want to welcome their baby into a lovely home that feels fresh and clean, which is why you might get sucked into all of those drab tasks you've been putting off for weeks. However, if you notice yourself verging on obsessive, this could be a positive sign that things are due to start happening. Think of it as you instinctively preparing your nest.

2. Cramping

A pretty universal description for the start of labour is a period-like, cramping feeling, often felt in the lower abdominals. If this is your only sign, it probably means that things are beginning to move along, and it's understandable that you may be uncertain about whether it really is time. Doubt often arises if the sensations are irregular, with a complete lack of intensity and no other accompanying signs. As you've seen from some of the previous birth stories, sometimes early labour can take a while.

Some will experience weak cramps for days or even weeks before they move into established labour, while for others things progress more quickly. If you experience cramping, look for consistency in the frequency of the sensations to indicate if early labour is starting. If you're destined to experience a long lead-up to labour, infrequent cramping sensations can be frustrating and confusing. This can be referred to as a long latent phase, or practice labour.

A good way to deal with the uncertainty is to practise the acceptance you'll be using while birthing: don't wish for things to hurry up, or think about when you're going to know for sure. If you're able to, go about your everyday business, staying as active as possible. If you can, get outside and go for a walk. Bear in mind when you're on the move that you might want to stay within an hour of your home, just in case. Continue to reassure yourself with the knowledge that your body is getting prepared. Sooner or later you'll be holding your baby in your arms, so relax and go with the flow.

3. Spotting

A little bit of light spotting – often partnered with the dislodging of the mucous plug (but not always) – is normal and a sign your body is preparing for labour and birth. If you notice any blood prior to 36 weeks or feel it is too heavy, it is always worth checking in with your medical care providers.

4. Waters releasing

This is one of the first signs that spring to mind for most people when we talk about indications for the onset of labour. Once again, a note about language: rather than talking about waters 'breaking', we encourage you to describe them as releasing. Nothing is broken during labour. It's all good.

What you might be surprised to learn is that the release of your waters isn't a given. You won't necessarily experience a big gush of liquid like you've probably seen in the movies. Sometimes this does happen, and it's not unusual to choose to sleep on towels, or have some type of protective covering for the mattress, just in case. Some will gush for hours on end; if this is you there is nothing to worry about – you're just releasing a lot of water.

However, many pregnant women and people find themselves unsure whether their waters have released at all, as they only feel dampness. We call this trickling. If you're a trickler, you're more likely to find yourself wondering whether you've wet yourself rather than if your waters have released. Sometimes you'll hear an audible pop when the waters release. Again, this is nothing to worry about.

In some cases your care providers will want you to travel to your place of birth to confirm whether your waters have released or not, and many will ask you to put on a sanitary towel so they can check for moisture and confirm the waters are clear and baby hasn't passed any meconium. Meconium is the equivalent of baby doing a poo in the amniotic sac and will turn your clear waters a shade of greeny-brown. It can sometimes – but certainly not always – be a sign that baby is in distress. Depending on your caregiver and the colour of the meconium, a general rule of thumb is the lighter the colour the happier your care providers will be. You will be asked to participate in continuous foetal monitoring, so your team can keep a close eye on baby's stress levels.

Other care providers are happy for you to stay at home and wait for you to travel until your surges are established. Speak to whomever you're working with in advance and find out what the protocol is so you can make appropriate plans for the big day.

5. Losing your mucous plug

Your mucous plug sits in the neck of your womb and as your cervix begins to get wider, this mucous membrane is discharged. Losing your mucous plug is a fantastic sign that your body is preparing for birth. However, be aware that this can happen up to two, or sometimes even three, weeks before you go into labour.

Your mucous plug can be clear and quite snotty-looking, but it can also be a bit pink in colour and sometimes look bloody. The loss of the mucous plug can sometimes be referred to as a 'bloody show', because the mucous becomes bloodstained. This is totally normal, and nothing to worry about.

6. Diarrhoea

We love a loose stool at The Calm Birth School! A bit of diarrhoea before or while you're experiencing early cramping sensations is a big green light that your body is expelling everything it needs to, making the path of descent as easy as possible for your baby. Bring on the poo!

7. Feeling nauseous or being sick

Nausea is another fantastic sign your body is doing what it needs to do and is clearing your digestive system so your body is in the optimal state for birthing.

Bonus sign: Intuition

You might sense you need to stay close to home on the day your labour begins. For example, it's not uncommon to hear of pregnant women or people saying even though they had no signs at all, they just knew that they should stay close to home that day.

How to deal with a long latent phase

The latent phase of labour is something that every birthing person experiences. It most commonly lasts 1–24 hours. While no latent phase is typical – everyone experiences it differently – a good indication you're experiencing the latent phase is getting non-regular surges or cramping. Surges can be very intense during the period and for some birthing women and people they are so mild that they don't even feel labour has begun.

For those who do feel intensity with their surges, this can be a challenging time as you just want to know when things are going to kick in properly, particularly if your irregular surges last longer than 24 hours. Yes. You read that correctly; the latent phase can last longer than 24 hours – we have had people looking for moral support after working with their body's surges for five days in the past! But of course this is where your Calm Birth School Method and your mindset come into play. Our top tips for not going insane during this period are as follows:

- Stay active for as long as feels humanly comfortable.

- Get down on all fours.

- Walk sideways up the stairs.

- Check out the website www.spinningbabies.com for more handy hints on positions you can take that may help to move baby into a more optimal position for birth.

- Look for support in the community group.

- Go for a massage or reflexology to help you relax.

- Appreciate that whatever happens you're going to be holding your baby in your arms for the first time soon enough.

- Listen to the audio downloads that most resonate with how you're feeling or where you would like your focus to be at the time.

- Remember to drink fluids.

- If you're feeling tired, it's totally OK to sleep.

- You know we love a fabulous warm bath too.

Expect to run the full range of emotions, happy and excited in the beginning to frustrated and angry and confused, the longer it goes on. All these emotions are totally normal. Acknowledge and look to release them as much as possible and focus on the fact that your body is preparing for your baby to meet you for the first time.

The main thing is to listen to your body.

What to do when labour starts

During the night

If your labour starts at night, rest, relax and conserve as much of your precious energy as possible. You don't want to feel tired just as your body and baby need you to feel energized. In the same vein, if your birth partner is with you and you go into labour at night, let your partner sleep if the sensations you're experiencing aren't very intense and you don't need support at this time. You'll want your partner to be as alert and supportive at the exact time you need them to be and if they're tired because they have been up for most of the time, that's going to be a problem. While there isn't any doubt that you've got the biggest job on the day, being a birth partner is a tiring job – even if all they appear to do is just sit and hold your hand.

Being in the early stages of labour when you would normally be asleep is one of the few times we would ever recommend you lying down. However, you can still do this with a slightly elevated back, by propping yourself up with cushions, or lie down on your side to create a more optimal position for baby.

During the day

If you're in early labour during the day, stay active but more importantly, always listen to your body and rest when you need to, in order to ensure you conserve your energy for when you most need it. When you feel a surge during early labour, stop moving and focus on your breath before continuing with your activities. Keep a 'business as usual' mindset. Stay active and keep your body as upright and forward as possible. This aids the natural process of working with gravity, helping to encourage your baby to stay in, or move into, the optimal position for birth. Look back to Chapter 10 (*see page 133*) for inspiration on how you and your birth partner can keep the vibe and those loving feelings oh, so high.

When it comes to chilling out, sitting down, bouncing on your birth ball and lying on your left side can all be great resting positions. One of your birth partner's roles will be to gently remind you to switch positions every 45 minutes or so. If they notice you have been static for too long, encouraging you to move will ensure you do everything you can to encourage baby to move down your birth path optimally.

If any part of you feels apprehensive instead of excited – and this counts during the daytime too – acknowledge the fears, practise your Calm Birth School breathing and release and let go of anything that is causing you anxiety. This will create the best foundation for a calm and comfortable birth.

℘ **Cat's abdominal birth story (twins)** ℘

Tuesday 9 March was my 36-week scan day. This scan was the decider. If twin one, Ivy, was still breech I was going to be having a scheduled abdominal birth. I was prepared for this situation, and Imogen, my TCBS Instructor, was a big part of that as leading up to this point I really didn't want an abdominal birth, mainly because of the recovery. BUT scan time arrived, the Doppler[52] was put on my ever-expanding tummy and guess what – both twins were head down! Hooray! Twin two, Willow, however, had dropped in weight quite significantly. The ultrasound technician and consultant weren't worried, so following that scan, the decision was made to cancel my scheduled section and pursue an induction on the same date.

Wednesday 10 March was my midwife appointment. Both girls' heart rates were lovely and they were both still nice and active in my tummy. Willow's weight was still in the back of my mind, however, so I queried it with my midwife, who then made an impromptu call to the consultant surgeon. It was then decided we would still go for the induction, but bring it forward a bit... to the next day! At 36+3 weeks' pregnant. To say I was shocked was an understatement. But I'd done all the lessons with Imogen, fortunately, and once again, thought, I am ready and prepared to deal with this.

On the morning of the planned induction, my husband John and I headed to the hospital. When we arrived, the midwife hooked me up to the CTG machine to check the girls' heart rates and the consultants scanned me to check the girls' placement. Both still head down and doing OK. The biggest concern at this point was whether my smaller twin would cope with an induction. Especially as it could take a few days to get me into labour – my due week was still another three weeks away. The choice was then up to me and John. Go for the induction or go for a scheduled abdominal birth? We chose the abdominal birth.

Around 1:45 p.m., my midwife came to collect me to go to theatre. This was it! Finally time to meet our girls. When I got into theatre my spinal anaesthetic was given and I was laid back on the operating table staring down at my bump for the final time. I used the visualization and breathing techniques taught to me by Imogen when my feelings started moving away from being calm, centred and focused. At 14:32 Ivy's head was delivered. The drapes were lowered and I saw my sweet daughter's face for the first time! A moment I will never forget! At 14:34 it was Willow's turn, once again the drapes were lowered and I saw my second daughter's head get delivered into the world and cry that sweet cry that every mama wants to hear. I don't know whether it was the head space I was in or the really good spinal anaesthetic, but I did not feel anything in terms of the caesarean being performed. No pulling or tugging. Completely numb.

Once both girls had received all the blood from their placentas, they were released from the cords and checked over by the baby doctors. Daddy – John – cut Ivy's cord and Mummy got to cut Willow's. It was then time for skin to skin. The calm I felt when my daughters were placed on my chest is like no other. Instant love and protectiveness washed over me and nothing mattered more in the world than them.

Imogen's class was one of the best things I could have joined in my pregnancy. I only wished I'd done it sooner. No matter what kind of birth you plan or end up having, it is 110 per cent designed for every woman/family and every birth! I definitely had a happy birth, so thank you Imogen from the bottom of my heart. ♥

∼

CHAPTER 14

Positions for Labour

W hen it comes to finding the best positions for birth, we urge you to follow your own natural birthing instincts and go with what feels comfortable. There are no rules as such, but there are certainly positions that can be more or less helpful for creating more positive birth experiences.

Active birthing: Sitting, squatting or on your hands and knees

Active birthing was made popular in the eighties through antenatal educator and birth pioneer, Janet Balaskas. After completing lots of her own research into birth in different cultures, it became increasingly clear that, far from being strapped down to beds and often anaesthetized, as was common in the West, in other cultures birthing women and people often kept moving while labouring until they felt ready and would then proceed to squat during the birthing phase. A study in 2012 finally provided supporting evidence that women who remained active and upright during birth had a significant decrease in interventions.[53]

Active birthing allows the pelvis to open, providing your baby with more space to travel through the birth path. There is also evidence that these types of positions lead to shorter labours.

Keeping mobile during active labour

The following positions will help you stay mobile and as relaxed as possible, in as optimal a position as possible, during labour.

- Sit down on the lavatory with your torso facing the cistern so you can rest your arms on the back of the toilet. This position can offer great relief alongside helping you open your pelvis.

- Sitting astride a chair, with your torso facing the backrest, can have the same effect as sitting on the loo.

- Hold on to your partner around their neck, while gently swaying or circling your hips.

- Sit on a birthing stool or chair or ball.

— **Tip** —

Check out www.thecalmbirthschool.com/bookbonuses for Katy Appleton from Apple Yoga's bonus video on prenatal yoga and different types of positions.

If possible, avoid lying on your back while you're labouring, as it will never help you birth your baby more quickly or comfortably. If you find yourself wanting to lie down on your back, discuss with your partner how they can help you stay mindful of moving around – without them sounding like they are ordering you about. Give yourself a limit of 30 minutes and then move into one of your favourite upright and forward positions.

When movement is more restricted

You may find yourself lying on your back if you need to have continuous monitoring or an epidural.

Continuous foetal monitoring may mean that you have to lie on your bed, so the machines can take as accurate a reading as possible. So before you get to this stage remember to use your BRAIN to identify if there are any other options available to you, like intermittent monitoring or wireless monitoring, so that you can still walk around, helping you to support your baby's descent more effectively.

When it comes to an epidural you may be thinking, what's the big deal, as I won't be able to feel anything? The impact of an epidural is less about comfort and more about the potential of you needing further assistance, as again, your pelvis will not be in the optimal position for guiding baby out into the world.

An alternative is to ask whether your care providers offer the option to have a low-dose epidural, which will still allow some feeling of sensations and may allow you to adopt a position on all fours for example. Alternatively, it is possible to ask that your epidural dosage be turned up and down, so you have more sensations when it is time to breathe your baby down. Both of these options can help to reduce the chances of you requiring a ventouse or a forceps delivery.

❧ **Elizabeth's birth story** ❧

Both my children have come fast – extremely fast. My experience with my first child was very traumatic for me, even though we were both healthy during and after the birth. I knew having my second child that it would also be a fast birth and I wanted to find a way to cope and make the birth a beautiful experience. I took a TCBS hypnobirthing course and it changed me as a mom and a woman in the best way possible. My instructor, Karis, gave me the support and tools that helped me prepare for the birth.

This birth didn't follow the 'standard' stages of labour. I lost my plug about a week before the birth. There were no Braxton Hicks contractions or any other signs. When I went for my due-date appointment at the hospital, they said it could happen anytime now. For a few days still nothing happened. Then, one morning I was feeling really tired so I went to lie down. I fell asleep and woke up to a pop feeling. My waters released. Then the surges hit hard and fast. I called the hospital to let them know I was on my way. I told them my surge times in hopes that I could have a water birth.

My husband and I rushed to the hospital. I used the breathing techniques all the way to the hospital. It was the only thing keeping me calm and not freaking out that I might just have this baby in the car. We arrived at the hospital. There was only one midwife available and she brought us into the delivery room. She took one quick look at me and said it's time to push. So 12 very intense minutes later my son was born and in my arms. We were both happy and healthy.

Those first few minutes were pure bliss looking at each other and cuddling. I didn't get the water birth I wanted, but it was still such a beautiful experience, it didn't matter. I felt in control this time. I was working with my body instead of against it. I listened to it with each push. I did the breathing practice I learned during the hypnobirthing course. I barely felt the pain of pushing and my son coming out. The breaths and the mindset helped me stay strong and present. It was such an incredibly positive and beautiful birth experience – I will look back on it and cherish it always.

CHAPTER 15

Active or Established Labour

Depending on where you are in the world, active labour is considered to begin from 5cm dilation onwards. Sometimes birthing women and people report they feel more intensity once established labour begins, some say as soon as they felt their first surge it was all systems go, and others report no difference between the early stages of labour or after they have surpassed the 5cm mark. Remember: everybody experiences labour and birth differently.

If you feel immense intensity straight away, rather than the gentle build-up many expect, remember you have all the tools you need to access a deep state of relaxation quickly. By simply using your Calm Birth School breathing (in for four and out for seven) followed by your wave breathing (in through the nose for seven and out through the mouth for seven) you won't need half an hour to enter a deep state of relaxation. You'll be able to access this state quickly and easily.

However, in order for this to come instinctively to you, you do need to practise breathing techniques regularly in situations non-conducive to relaxation. Don't wait until it's late at night and you're all warm and cosy in bed to practise. Go for it when you're in the middle of chaos, being bumped about on public transport, or wanting to explode at your birth partner because they have said the wrong thing... again. When this happens, your body will become used to responding with relaxation once you step into the less-familiar territory of giving birth.

When to travel to your care provider

If you're birthing outside your home, the closer you are to established labour, the less likely it is you'll need any medical intervention. For first-time birthers, I recommend that unless you're going to feel safer or more comfortable travelling to your place of birth earlier, stay at home until you experience four waves in 10 minutes, each lasting for about a minute, consistently for two hours. For those of you who have done this before, three waves in 10 minutes, lasting between 45 seconds to a minute, is a good rule of thumb.

> ## — Tip —
>
> If your birth partner is with you, let them time and measure the frequency of your waves.

Some birthing women and people prefer not to use a clock to time their waves for a valid reason: whenever we engage with something that requires us to use our rational mind, it is more difficult to distance ourselves from the sensations we are experiencing in our bodies. Having your birth partner in control of the clock can help if you're going down this route. Having some kind of signal or trigger word so they know when to start and stop the timer can also minimize chatting if you're the type of person who prefers to focus all their energy inwards when they are birthing. Maybe you'll be extremely engaged and talkative in between surges and, until you get to the day, you simply don't know which camp you'll fall into, so it's useful to have a plan.

An alternative method for measuring how far dilated you are comes from the book *The Art of Midwifery* by Hilary Marland and utilizes the fact the body is diverting more blood away from the legs and feet towards the uterus in order to increase its efficiency while we are birthing. When a birthing woman or person is 1–2cm dilated, the feet and ankles are colder; once she reaches 3–5cm, the calves are colder; and then at full dilation of 10cm, the legs are cold from the knee downwards. Clever, right? Be aware that this isn't a technique you can use if you have been getting in and out of the shower or bath, since the warm water will change your body temperature.

> ## — Tip —
>
> If you're birthing at home, talk to your care provider about when would be the best time during the process for you to contact them before they come to you.

Whenever you experience a surge, use your Calm Birth Method breathing techniques to eliminate tension in the body. Then move into your wave breathing, aiming for equal length inhalations and exhalations. Ideally, your body will be as limp as possible, like a rag doll, so there is no resistance in your mind or your body.

When you call your care providers, often they will want to talk directly to you as the birthing person, as they like to listen to how you're breathing and to assess how the waves are affecting your ability to speak. Let them know you're using hypnobirthing, as it's likely you'll be managing the normal stress and intensity of labour much more effectively than they will anticipate, leading to some care providers to conclude you're not as far along as you really are. Make sure you monitor the frequency of surges and communicate this to them.

How long will you be in labour for?

The answer to this question is: how long is a piece of string? Some people will pop their bambinos out in a few short hours, others will be closer to 40, 50 and sometimes even 60 hours. And I have encountered both ends of the spectrum with students who have used The Calm Birth Method.

The one thing that sets students of The Calm Birth Method aside from non-hypnobirthers is even if you're in labour for a LONG time, you can use the tools and techniques you have been practising to help you transform what, for some birthing women and people, is a difficult and challenging time into something that helps you feel powerful and in control as you enjoy your labouring experience.

CHAPTER 16

Coping with Distractions

I f you're choosing to birth in your own environment, it's much easier to feel comfortable about managing the potential distractions around you. When you know you'll be moving from your home to a birthing centre or a hospital, there are inevitably more distractions you'll encounter along the way, many of which you will not be able to do anything about. I want to reassure you that outside distractions don't need to be the end of your positive birth experience. You're a master at filtering out distractions in your everyday life and we will be tapping into this awesome skill of yours in the lead-up to, and on the big day itself.

The brain processes 400 billion pieces of information every second, of which we are aware of around 2,000. Then we filter out the things we deem unimportant or irrelevant to what is going on in our surroundings. This filtering method stops us from going insane. Thank you, nature! This mechanism is precisely why you don't need to get your knickers in a twist about being distracted. It is also the exact same mechanism I want you to tap into when you're birthing. You can start practising it right now. In fact you already are, but perhaps aren't fully conscious of it yet.

Your guide for when to consciously tune in to this filter and when not to is really simple. If you're faced with a situation that is creating tension or irritation within you and it's something you can do something about, (a dripping tap or a snoring partner, for example), then do something about it. Take charge; these situations can be remedied quickly and easily.

If, however, you're faced with a tension-inducing situation that you do not have the power to change, choose instead to focus your attention inwards and start to watch and engage with your breath using The Calm Birth School breathing techniques (surprise, surprise!). Allow the distraction to take you even deeper into a state of relaxation. You can even say to yourself, 'The sound of [*insert distraction*] helps me drift deeper and deeper into a beautiful state of relaxation.' A great time to play with this is when your baby is having a kick and a stretch while you're doing your daily relaxation exercises. Any time there is intrusive noise or something happening within your line of sight, use it as an opportunity to connect to your breath consciously.

This will be easier or harder to do depending on the distraction, but the more you practise, the easier it will become. A great example is when someone else's child is crying on a plane. Some people will be there wishing they were in the peace and quiet of Business Class, while others will be able to fall asleep in the midst of chaos, appearing completely undisturbed. Your opportunity to practise might come on a bus or train, while waiting for an appointment, or perhaps when you're at a family gathering. The aim, by the time you go into labour, is for you to be a person who can choose exactly when and where you want to focus your attention, and who can breathe through anything.

By making the conscious decision to focus on your breath and allow the distraction to help you go deeper into relaxation, you can change the whole experience of the noises around you with ease. This is a skill that takes practice, but you can do it. The trick is to start, so I encourage you to make a start today.

Positive power of touch

To help manage the internal distractions – i.e. your waves – take advantage of the positive power of touch.

Touch is an important part of intimacy between couples, as it helps them to relax, feel connected and safe. All these emotions are great for producing endorphins and oxytocin, which we now know are the ones we want for a quicker, more comfortable labour (as opposed to cortisol and adrenaline). We recommend that you and your partner make time to really tune in to this during pregnancy by enjoying daily massage with each other – and, when we say each other, I mean the birth partner massaging the pregnant half of the couple! Some people will enjoy a firm pressure, but the massage I recommend involves a very light touch.

However, it is also worth noting that, even after taking the time to enjoy this fantastic ritual during pregnancy, when you're labouring you might not want anyone within an inch of you! Some birthers have reported they needed to be alone so they went and birthed in the bathroom. That's also absolutely fine. Massage is an extra tool you can call upon should you want it on the day, and it will be infinitely more powerful if you take the time during your pregnancy to really connect a sense of calm to your partner's touch.

Massage

The light touch of this massage technique often creates a tingly feeling within the body and is simple to use.

How to do it

Your partner or birth partner uses their fingertips or the backs of the fingernails in a gentle upward motion, stroking and moving their fingers up your back and across your shoulders, almost creating a T-shape. Repeat and then repeat some more.

You can also bring these soothing strokes up and down the arms, across the chest and nipples, up the neck, behind the ears and into the hair. This is definitely a useful tool to draw upon if labour slows down.

When to do it

A daily 15-minute massage is ideal, as this is not only a great way to build on your opportunity for prenatal bonding, but the touch of the birth partner becomes a cue or an anchor for you to become even more relaxed every time this type of touch occurs, which can be extremely valuable during labour.

Dial Down Method

Another great method for distancing yourself from both internal and external distractions is the Dial Down Method, which is a self-hypnosis tool. This is a great tool to use whenever you notice yourself feeling tense or stressed and you have a little bit of time on your hands. It's the perfect technique to draw upon if you're on public transport, or when travelling.

How to do it

Imagine a large dial, with the numbers one to 10 going around the perimeter. As you imagine the dial, see the gauge hovering at number 10.

Then take a deep breath in, imagine breathing in calm and as you exhale, imagine breathing out tension. On the completion of that exhalation, see the gauge move to the number nine. Again, inhale calm and exhale tension, then see the gauge move down to eight.

Do this all the way to zero and you should notice how much more relaxed your mind and body feel. When you get to zero you can continue to focus your attention on the breath, or imagine relaxing in your favourite place. Play with it and follow your gut instinct.

You can amend this technique and visualize a big temperature gauge, a sliding scale of musical notes or a thermometer – whatever makes the most sense to you.

When to do it

Most people start practising this visualization with their eyes closed, but as soon as you become familiar with it, eyes open is equally effective. If you're ever in the office, particularly if you're in one of those meetings – you know the ones I'm talking about – and need to get out of your head for a bit, this is a great trick to have up your sleeve.

When TCBS students first start using this technique, it doesn't always come naturally. Many of the techniques I've shared may feel difficult to get your head around at first. Please persevere and be kind to yourself. It is the same when you learn any new skill – it takes time and a lot of repetition to master any new practice to a point where you can do it on autopilot.

Think about when you learned to ride a bike or drive a car, or a toddler trying to find their walking legs: how many times will you see them pull themselves up, only to topple over? It's all part of the learning process, and it takes time, effort and perseverance. It's exactly the same with the skills you're learning throughout this book too, which is why I recommend starting now, not a couple of weeks before your guess date!

. . . .

Time distortion

Hypnobirthing birthers often talk about the quickening of the passage of time when they are birthing, and this is a noticeable indication of being in a trance state. It's similar to being engrossed in a great book – you have just no idea where the time went. You can have the exact same experience during birth of time working with or against you, depending on how you're feeling in the moment.

Time flies for someone who feels relaxed and calm and looks forward to each surge, as an indication that each sensation brings them one step closer to meeting their baby. Contrast this with someone who dreads every surge and wonders when it's finally going to be over and how long labour is going to last. Every minute feels like 10... or more.

When you feel good, your birth partner can capitalize on this sense of time passing more quickly, by suggesting every 20 minutes feels like five. While it might feel silly reading this right now, remember that when you're birthing you're going to be in a trance state and therefore more open to suggestion, so use that in your favour.

ಶಿ **Claudia's birth story** ಶಿ

I started to plan my birth and write my birth preferences – I'd always dreamt of a home water birth, although having chatted through the pros and cons with my husband Benjamin, due to our past experiences he felt nervous about this. So we both decided together that having our baby at The Bluebell Centre at Warwick Hospital would be the best option for us, although as I was 'high-risk' this wasn't a possibility. All was going well with my pregnancy and baby was growing perfectly. Hypnobirthing gave me the confidence to ask the right questions, and so at my next consultant appointment I was discharged from high-risk care and transferred over to the care of a midwife.

My hospital bag was packed, birth preferences were printed, cool box for my placenta was waiting by the door. All I had to do was wait patiently for my baby. I was feeling hot, uncomfortable and needed to wee every time I walked, as baby was so low. Because Maddox (my son) had arrived at 37w 2d this was the most pregnant I'd ever been and I just wanted my baby here safely. I had acupuncture, reflexology, massage, diffused Clary Sage aromatherapy oils and insisted my husband do his 'duty' to help baby along – but nothing.

Then on the morning of Tuesday 9 July, two days before my estimated due date, I was casually eating breakfast with my mum, Benjamin and Maddox while sat on my birthing ball and felt as though I needed the toilet again with a little pressure on my back passage. I went to the toilet and got into the shower as thought I'd get washed/ dressed in case it was my labour starting. While in the shower I started having more sensations, stronger this time, and I knew it was my baby! I measured the surges and they were immediately two minutes apart – time to go!

Luckily my in-laws arrived just in time to look after Maddox, so I made my way to the car, managing my surges with my breathing techniques – which were very intense by this point. Finally in the passenger seat, my intuition kicked in and I just knew I wouldn't get to hospital on time. Then my waters released and I could feel pressure moving down. I asked Benjamin to remove my knickers and instead of pulling them down, he ripped them off like a caveman and threw them on the drive :0)

The ambulance service were on the phone talking him through things and asking questions about my condition, people started to panic and I was aware of things becoming out of control. I completely blocked out the panic, took myself into my hypnobirthing practice – especially my breathing – and visualized my baby arriving safely, holding him/her in my arms. Intuitively, I knew that I wouldn't make it to the Bluebell Centre and there was no way I was having my baby in the car, so I asked Benjamin to help me back into my living room. Once there, I flopped down onto my rug on all fours, hugged my birthing ball and breathed through my extremely intense surges. I could hear the ambulance service giving Benjamin instructions and someone ran off to get towels, but I was completely in my zone of calm and relaxation, even though everyone was panicking.

Just 12 minutes after my waters had released I felt the urge to breathe my baby down, along with stretching sensations, and baby's head was born. One more deep long breath down and Benjamin caught baby in a towel. Baby wasn't making any noise and while Benjamin rubbed them with the towel it felt like an eternity. Then I heard them cry – such relief! In all the excitement he announced it was a boy, then I heard my mother-in-law screaming, 'It's a girl!' I think my response was, 'Well, which is it?!' Then my beautiful, perfect, healthy baby girl was placed on my chest to breastfeed. I was overcome with love and still in my relaxed, calm bubble holding my little girl!

Two ambulance crews arrived four minutes later and checked us both over. The umbilical cord had stopped pulsating by this point so it was clamped (a little longer so that we could use our umbilical cord tie later) and Benjamin cut the cord. While I focused on delivering my placenta naturally, Daddy enjoyed skin to skin with his little girl, Maddox got to meet his little sister and she got to meet her nana, nanny and grandad.

Unfortunately, my placenta wasn't really moving, so we were taken to Warwick Hospital by ambulance to be checked over properly. I was still so very relaxed, calm and couldn't quite believe I was holding my beautiful baby. Luckily, when the midwife checked, my placenta was naturally ready to be delivered and was checked/ put on ice ready to be collected by the lady doing my placenta encapsulation.

Due to how quickly baby arrived, I had to have some stitches, which I felt completely relaxed about. We were just enjoying cuddles with our new bundle, laughing and chatting. I didn't feel as though I had just given birth; in fact, I felt amazing!

Marnie is so calm; she breastfeeds amazingly (constantly), sleeps well and is definitely a relaxed hypnobirthing baby! I'm very lucky and know that hypnobirthing has yet again given me another amazing birth experience! I wish I could do it all over again!

≈

CHAPTER 17

What Happens Once You're with Your Care Provider?

Once there is space for you on the labour ward or in your room – if you're not birthing at home – most of the time you'll be offered a vaginal examination. Note the use of the word 'offered'. A vaginal examination, as with all procedures offered during birth, is provided on informed consent, so it is your right to decline a vaginal examination should you wish to.

Why would you decline this? Well, some birthers want to have a completely undisturbed birth and believe baby will arrive whenever they are ready. Their perspective is that a vaginal examination does nothing to aid that process. It's also recognized that a VE only measures a moment in time. So, if you go to the hospital, are examined and a well-meaning midwife says, 'Oh, you're only 2cm,' the use of the word 'only', plus the fact that you're 2cm, can be hugely deflating. If you do opt for an examination, remember that it is just a moment in time, labour isn't linear and things can progress very quickly.

I can't emphasize this enough: if you opt for a vaginal examination – and many do – and you're not progressing as quickly as you would like, relax and do as many oxytocin- and endorphin-producing activities as possible.

This really is your birth partner's time to shine and remind you, you birthing beauty, that this is just a moment in time and you're doing amazingly. Just because it's taken 10 hours to reach 3cm, doesn't mean it's going to take another 10 hours to get to 6cm. When you're relaxed and birthing as actively as possible, it's not uncommon to go from 3cm to 8cm in an hour! This is, in fact, exactly what happened to Liz in her third birth!

If you find that you haven't progressed at the rate you would have liked, know that it's totally normal to feel frustrated and concerned about how much longer things are going to take and then consciously choose to release the expectation or the wish for things to be different. Let go of any tension, doubt or anxiety that may be trying to creep in and simply be accepting of the moment.

This isn't easy to do if you haven't been practising breathing and sending relaxation to the different parts of your body, both at home and in less conducive places for relaxation, such as on public transport. So make sure you practise in advance!

The slowdown

Whether you're travelling to a hospital or birthing at home, it's very common at one point or another during your labour for things to slow down. Depending on what stage you decide to leave home, if you do at all, a slowdown occurs because you're leaving your cosy and familiar home environment. This is normal and all part of the evolutionary armoury that aims to keep us and our babies safe from harm while our subconscious assesses the reasons we have moved and whether it feels good to continue with the labour.

If your body and baby decide to take a little break, you might like to use one or more of the following ideas to help get your surges going again:

1. **Breathing techniques:** You'll have practised these so many times by this point that your muscle memory associates breathing with feeling good, being calm and at ease, which acts as a signal for you to produce more endorphins and oxytocin.

2. **Touch:** Remember the power of positive touch, whether it is a little bit of massage, stroking or holding. If you feel open to being held or touched, give your birth partner the green light, if they have not already taken their cue.

3. **Walking:** Walk upstairs while leaning forward to help baby put more pressure on your cervix. Walking sideways upstairs can also help – think like a crab!

4. **Visualization:** See your baby moving down the birth path and how good it's going to feel to be holding them in your arms, or listen to your Birth Rehearsal audio download – all roads lead to oxytocin.

5. **Nipple stimulation:** This is great if things slow down as the stimulation of the nipples impacts the body in a similar way to when a baby is suckling, causing the body to produce oxytocin to help promote bonding and attachment. Of course oxytocin production will increase the efficiency of your labour.

6. **Laughter:** Watch anything that makes you laugh. Download it to your device beforehand so you've got easy access to it. We laugh when we're relaxed, and when we're relaxed, we birth babies more quickly, easily and comfortably. Trust that your body and your baby know what to do and things will pick up again at exactly the right time. The best thing you can do is relax.

7. **A warm bath:** Water can either speed labour up, or slow things down, so it's wise to be mindful. If you're experiencing irregular surges that slow down after you have hit the water, get out. However, the flip side of that is the lovely warm water stimulating your oxytocin and endorphins, and helping things along beautifully.

Best avoided

While I think films (hilarious ones) are a great idea, mobile phones, laptops or anything that will engage the rational, analytical part of your brain should be banned during birth if you're looking to create a quicker and more comfortable birthing experience.

And certainly, no to social media once you're in active labour: no tweeting, no posting on Insta, Facebook or texting your friends. The more you disengage from the left side of your brain – the part responsible for critical analysis – the easier you'll find it to connect with the sensations in your body, rather than analyse them from a cognitive distance.

It's also worth thinking about whether you want to let anyone know once things have started to get going, because if you're going to experience a longer labour, the pressure of having people texting you or your birth partner to find out what is happening can also create unnecessary stress, pressure or analytical engagement.

Working with your care provider during labour

Ensure you have at least two copies of your birth preferences with you, so if there is a change of shift when you're birthing, your new care provider can get up to speed.

As we have discussed, who you have in the birthing room is hugely important and your birth partner should be responsible for managing your environment, so highlight this section for your birth partner to read.

It is the birth partner's role to be fully tuned in to the person who is birthing, so they can see how you are feeling and talk to the people who are working for you. Please remember they are working for you. If there is any hint your practitioners aren't supportive, or there is a personality clash, your partner needs to take the lead and, in a calm, but firm way, ask for you to be cared for by someone else. It isn't your responsibility to be concerned about how that is managed, but it is your partner's responsibility to hold and protect the space, so that you have an optimal birthing environment, which is full of peace, love and support. Then you'll be able to make the decisions that are right for you and your family.

Remember, you'll only have this experience once. So you have to make the choice about whether it's best to be more concerned with ensuring that you create the most positive birth experience for you and your family or worry about potentially offending someone who is unable to support you in the way that you need in that moment... I know what I'd choose.

Decide beforehand whether you would like your birth partner to act as a go-between for you and your care providers when it comes to making decisions about the birth, or whether you would like to take the lead. As always there are no rights or wrongs when it comes to this, but if you're looking to birth more comfortably and quickly, the less you engage in conversation, the better.

Many hospitals will want to see progression of about 1cm dilation per hour. But you're not a machine, so often it does not work like this. Once again it's important for your birth partner to be tuned in to how you're feeling so they can alleviate any pressure you may encounter from people trying to speed things up.

If you find yourself in a situation where people are trying to hurry things along, use the BRAIN system and ask very specific questions. This will provide you with specific answers and allow you to make informed and personal choices about the course of action that is right for you. Always bring any suggestions about proceeding back to the specific indications at that moment, and be as specific as you can.

Example questions

- What specific evidence suggests that there will be a risk of [*insert complication*] happening?

- What specific signs right now indicate that waiting for the next 30 minutes would be harmful to me or my baby?

- If we choose to wait another 45 minutes, what are the possible risks, and what evidence do you have that those risks are applicable to my baby and me?

Language

By this point, I hope you're being mindful of the language you're using (*see page xxv*) to think and talk about birth. I've talked at length throughout this book about using different terminology and being very mindful of the kind of thoughts you think. Unfortunately, you can't control the words used by others. That said, it wouldn't do you any harm to include how you would like your care providers to talk to you in terms of comfort levels and waves, as opposed to pain and contractions, in your birth preferences.

- Certain words and phrases used by the medical profession can be upsetting or even distressing to hear during labour. Prepare yourself in advance by making a note of the terms below and making a decision about what you and your birth partner will do if you notice this language during your birth.

- For example, if someone in your space is using negative language, it is totally acceptable for the birth partner to respectfully ask the care provider to speak with them directly first, quietly and even outside the room if possible. The birthing environment should be kept as emotionally safe and relaxed as possible.

Some common phrases that are often used are as follows:

- **Failure to progress:** If you happen to hear this when you're labouring, remember that you always have options about whether you would like to follow the lead of your body, or if you would appreciate some assistance. Once again, go back to your BRAIN and assess what you feel is going to be right for you.

- **Incompetent contractions:** Whoa! Incompetent is definitely another phrase that should be banned from birthing rooms. There is nothing incompetent about your body and sometimes, for good reasons, your baby will stop moving down the birth path and you'll require assistance. It might simply mean that you need to move around, change positions and take the pressure off in order to allow the oxytocin to do the job it was designed to do.

- **You're only [*insert number*] centimetres dilated:** This is a HUGE no-no in my book. Dilation ONLY measures a moment in time. As we've seen, just because it took you three hours to get to 4cm, it doesn't mean it's going to take you another three hours to get to 8cm. Please include in your birth preferences, that if you choose to ask for an update, your care providers should frame your progress with encouragement, like 'You're doing well; you're currently X cm.' Or, 'This is where we are at right now.'

- **How much pain are you in?** While we don't ban the P word, it's much more helpful for your care team to ask, 'How comfortable are you?'

- **You're not allowed:** It doesn't matter what this is in reference to, quite frankly it's not true. It's your baby and your body, so if you want something to happen, you're entitled to have it happen.

- **We are going to...** Informed consent is required for all interventions, treatments and procedures. Always feel entitled to ask questions if someone looks to be moving forward with something you don't understand or agree with.

With any decisions you make about how involved you would like your care providers to be, remember that you have a choice.

If you opt for support to move things along a little, and make these decisions while feeling calm and in control, you remove any ambiguity because you can ask specific questions and receive specific answers. This contributes hugely to you being able to look back on your experience knowing you had the right birth for you, regardless of how your baby entered into the world. That can only be a positive thing.

Things to be mindful of during the active phase include:

- changing positions and keeping as active as possible

- using positive touch and words for comfort and reassurance

- making your birthing environment – particularly if you're not birthing at home – as lovely and as nest-like as possible

- having your birth partner hold the birthing space so it feels calm, private and safe.

CHAPTER 18

Second-Stage Labour

You're considered to be fully dilated at 10cm, sometimes referred to as the 'down phase' or 'second stage of labour'. It means your baby is close to being ready to emerge. There are three main factors to be aware of, which I'll talk you through now.

The three signs of second-stage labour

For many, the second stage of labour can mean an increase in intensity, although this isn't always the case.

A pause

At this point, just as during early labour, the body may take a natural break as it and your baby instinctively prepare for this new phase. This isn't the same as the slowdown (see Chapter 17, page 192), and it's nothing to worry about or hurry, as long as your baby's heartbeat is strong and consistent. Sometimes, this pause will be 10 minutes – and I've even heard stories of the break lasting a few hours.

If you're birthing at home with an independent or private midwife, it is far more likely they will feel comfortable going with the body's lead at this point. If you're birthing in a more medicalized environment, it's more likely that your care team will want to move things along if the break is deemed to be too long. If you're faced with this scenario, remember to use the BRAIN system to determine what course of action is going to be best for you and your family, and to make sure you're clear as to why any suggestions are being made (*see also Chapter 10, page 134*).

Sometimes, instead of a pause, you might notice an increase of intensity or frequency in the waves you're experiencing, or perhaps a change in the sensation of the surges. Everyone's experience is different.

Pooing

Many pregnant women and people fear doing a poo while bearing down in labour, and sh*t does happen (sometimes), but remember that it's all for our own good. Once you move into the second phase, the body's primary focus is to work as efficiently as it can and so it expels anything that may inhibit the baby from moving along the birth path. As the baby moves past the bowel, any waste is emptied to leave the birth path as clear as possible and thus make the baby's descent easier.

So, should you start to feel an overwhelming urge to do a poo, be happy, because it means that you're in the second stage and close to meeting your baby. Sometimes you might feel the urge to do a poo, but not actually end up doing one. This is great too. It simply means that baby is moving down the birth path, but that you don't have any waste to expel.

If you feel the need to do a poo once you're fully dilated, resist the urge to jump up and go to the toilet if you can, and move your attention back to your breath. It's time to begin breathing your baby down. If you're not participating in vaginal examinations, trust yourself to know that things are changing and you're moving into the second phase. Some people may call this the 'pushing phase'.

For some it will feel as though the body is taking over and for others, it will be a more conscious decision to change the way they are breathing with their surges. At this point, I invite you to choose to focus your energy and your breath downwards, working with your body and assisting your baby's journey.

Feeling nauseous

Another great indication you're moving into the second phase is vomiting or feeling nauseous. You could find yourself projectile-vomiting across the room after a substantial period of labour, accompanied by an increase in either the frequency or intensity of your surges. Alternatively, you may notice your surges dying off as your body pauses before you prepare to cross the final hurdle. There's no one direct route – it's all positive!

Pushing and breathing

When we watch people giving birth on TV, the second stage is what we usually associate with lots of forced pushing, and care providers shouting and coaching the birthing mother or person. Some of you may want the support of your midwives, and others may prefer quiet to let the body do what it innately knows how to do. As always, nature thinks of everything and, as for every other birthing mammal, there is no need to force your baby out. Your body has a unique mechanism for doing this on your behalf, called the natural expulsive reflex. You'll already be familiar with it from using it whenever you go for a poo.

Breathing baby down

When you're in this downward phase, the best thing you can do to aid this process is imagine sending your breath and energy down into the ground, past your baby, around your uterus and into the floor. This allows your body, pelvis and vagina to be as relaxed and open as possible for a quicker and more comfortable birth.

Some women experience an overwhelming urge to push or bear down. If this is you, I advise you to go for it. Listen to your body; do not resist it, even if 15 minutes previously you were told you were 'only' 6cm dilated. As mentioned earlier, vaginal examinations only measure a moment in time, and things can change very quickly. Trust your body.

So what's the difference between pushing and bearing down – if your body is telling you to do so – and forced or coached pushing? In a word: tension.

What I'd like you to do, either when you're sitting on the lavatory or sitting in your chair right now, is to pretend that you're pushing out a poo. What do you notice? You should feel the muscles around your sphincter contract and tighten – which is the exact opposite of the action we are looking for with a calm and positive birth for both you and your baby. When you can breathe your baby down and work with your body, your baby tends to make their entrance in a calmer, less explosive way, which also helps to keep the perineum intact. Bonus.

Having said that, for a multitude of reasons, some birthers will opt to force-push their babies into the world. As with every piece of advice or insight I offer throughout this book, if this is a conscious decision, coming from you, then it's all good. If you're faced with a situation that dictates that forced pushing is the best way forward and it feels right for you, then it's right. I really want you to hear me on this: you can't get this wrong. Just go with what feels right for you on the day.

Birth breathing

Use this technique when you're experiencing a wave or surge when you're fully dilated.

How to do it

The best way to aid the natural expulsive reflex is to work with the breath in a similar way to when you're wave breathing (*see Chapter 3, page 44*). The main difference is that you place all the emphasis on the exhalation; the out-breath needs to be very long and very deep. It can be useful to use a visualization to accompany the out-breath – anything that reminds you of the importance of staying open, relaxed and moving downwards.

Some people use the words 'open', 'relaxed' or 'release', others will think about there being no resistance, or imagine a flower opening, or will picture something significant to them that helps keep the idea of openness in their minds.

It can be really helpful to work with noise when you're getting to this stage. Although some will feel equally comfortable working with the breath alone, others will want to hum, shout, groan or even moo. If it hasn't already, it can get incredibly primal at this stage. This is nothing to be fearful of, for either you or your birth partner. No resistance is the main aim of the game. If you want to howl, just howl! Whatever you instinctively want to do is all good – seriously. The only thing to be mindful of is to use the noise and the energy to send your power back down to your baby and your uterus so they can finish the job.

When to do it

The best place to practise this technique is when you're having a poo. If you're at home, hum when you're on the loo so you start to feel more comfortable and familiar with directing your sound and energy down in that way.

This is great if you're suffering with constipation too. It won't shift everything immediately but by applying patience, the humming and breathing will see your natural expulsive reflex start to get things moving much more quickly and comfortably.

CHAPTER 19

Transition and Crowning

There often comes a moment during birth when a birthing woman or person thinks, 'I can't do this any more!'

The second phase usually lasts a maximum of two hours – although this will vary from person to person. Sometimes, right before baby is about to emerge, a birthing person may feel overwhelmed, like they can't do it any more and want to give up. This is called the transition stage. If this happens to you, this is an amazing sign for you and your birth partner that you're now within spitting distance (excuse the analogy!) of meeting your baby.

This is the time for your birth partner to remind you of what an amazing woman or person you are, and let you know you have reached the final hurdle. This period of wanting to give up or feeling like it's all too much right before the prize doesn't happen to everyone. However, if it does happen, take peace in the knowledge it is only likely to last for around 15 minutes, and you really are going to be meeting your baby at any moment.

Once the transition phase has passed (if you experience it at all), the last moments of birth are all about you working with your body to breathe baby into the world. Just as baby is about to emerge, you may experience an intense tingling sensation. This is your baby stretching and pulling on the vaginal walls, otherwise known as crowning. This intensity only lasts for a short time and is often followed by numbness, so aim to stay relaxed. Sometimes, the sensation of your baby's head crowning can come as a shock – as crazy as it may sound don't be tempted to close your legs (it does happen)! Focus on your birth breathing and waiting for the next surge to breathe out your baby's head fully, which should then be followed by their body, in just two to three surges.

✍ Tara's birth story ✍

I just wanted to let you know that our twins arrived last week and I was able to have my second amazing hypnobirthing birth. I was absolutely petrified about getting induced early (as it was twins). As I'd had a short water birth with my first, I think I was scared of the unknown and all the planned intervention as it was twins. But I was very lucky and my waters went just a few hours after the first pessary, and labour came on thick and fast. I was on my own for the three hours it took to become fully dilated (I appreciate I was very lucky with that) on the induction ward, which was overwhelmed by lots of people progressing quickly at once and didn't allow partners to stay. This made me even more scared, as I could hear everyone labouring in what sounded like a lot of pain around me and I was afraid of facing that on my own if it escalated to that.

I tried to embrace my inner Liz, and stay calm and breathe through each surge counting each breath in and out. Music and relaxation breathing really helped for the few light surges I had before my waters went, but afterwards, I just had to focus on the breathing to get through each one. Well, it worked – maybe too well, as I was so calm (and a bit too quiet), no one on the ward monitored the babies until I was fully dilated! Cue a lot of panic trying to get me to delivery and for them to assemble the 'twin' team. I said on the trolley that the consultant had wanted me to have an epidural in case twin two struggled, and asked whether they give that to me now. I said I didn't really want it, as I was scared it would stop things. They just laughed at me and first twin was born 15 minutes later. My husband only made the birth with five minutes to go! So ladies, don't underestimate hypnobirthing; if you feel like you're getting closer, press the buzzer!

CHAPTER 20

Your Baby's Here!

Even though many a wise parent will tell you that the real work begins once baby arrives, there's a little bit in between giving birth and starting parenting that is worth thinking about and preparing for.

Those moments when you hold your precious baby for the first time are not only magical because you're getting to look into each other's eyes, but also because you start to close the complex physiological and emotional loop of birth.

Cleaning your baby

If your baby is born on dry land, as opposed to in the water, you'll notice a white coating on your baby's skin. This is called 'vernix'. Some people prefer their baby to be completely wiped down before enjoying skin to skin with their child; others prefer things to be left au naturel. The choice is yours. However, some will argue that babies aren't born dirty and the rush to clean them just isn't necessary; vernix acts as an antiseptic moisturizer for baby's skin and protects them from a whole host of infections.

Delayed cord clamping

Delayed cord clamping is when the umbilical cord isn't cut immediately. Some parents are happy to leave it for two minutes before cutting, while others prefer to wait until the cord has stopped pulsating completely before cutting, so they know baby has everything they need from the placenta.

One of the things you can research is whether delayed cord clamping will be suitable for you or not. As you've read in some of the stories from TCBS students throughout this book, the idea of delayed cord clamping might seem perfect for you, until you actually go into labour, when circumstances can change very quickly.

If this is of interest, please do your own research into the benefits and drawbacks of this course of action, and be mindful your choice is very important to include on your birth preferences sheet.

Birthing your placenta

Birthing your placenta is one of those things that for some people can come as a total shock (*ahem, that would be me – Liz – and me – Suzy!*). We spend all of our time preparing to stay calm, relaxed and in control for our babies. Once we finally get to welcome them into the world, it can sometimes feel like a bit of a shock to realize the job isn't over yet. If you have been giving birth in a pool, you may be asked to get out and birth your placenta on dry land. And while some placentas plop out without having to give it a second thought, sometimes it takes a little bit of effort. If you're at the end of the spectrum that requires a little bit of focus, remember that all the skills you applied to birth your baby can be just as relevant for this third and final stage.

It is worth researching whether you would like to have a managed third stage when birthing your placenta, or whether you would prefer to let the process take its natural course. If you have a managed third stage, you'll receive an injection of synthetic oxytocin to stimulate the uterus into surging. This often means the third stage is over within half an hour. A managed third stage is often recommended, as it tends to reduce the numbers of those experiencing a large loss of blood after birthing. One of the disadvantages of taking a synthetic drug to speed up the process is that it increases the chances of retaining parts of your placenta,[54,55] which can lead to infection and sickness.[56] Once again, do your own research so you can decide which option is right for you.

If you opt to just let your placenta emerge on its own, it is worth putting this on your birth preferences because in some parts of the world consent to use the drug is sought when the baby's head is emerging. This could mean you end up saying yes, when you planned to say no! A physiological placenta delivery is assisted by encouraging that old friend of ours... yes, oxytocin. Skin to skin (*see below*) and eye contact with baby will help with this no end. As will breastfeeding/chestfeeding or just having baby close to your chest. Often when a baby is born, the lights go on, the attention goes straight to baby, the noise increases and you know as well as I do now that oxytocin does not thrive in that environment! You'll need privacy, dim lighting and to feel comfortable. Adopt a position that feels good to you (upright positions will help with gravity).

If you want a middle ground to the above, you could consider delaying the injection and wait for the cord to stop pulsating. While this happens your birth partner can step in and ensure that the environment is suitable and that you have the opportunity to encourage the natural release of oxytocin.

If labour is induced, a managed delivery of the placenta will be advised because the drugs used during an induction will inhibit the natural release of oxytocin.

Skin to skin

Skin to skin – the act of placing your baby directly on your exposed upper body/chest area either immediately, or as soon as possible, after birth – is one of nature's most awesome design features. Creating the space to allow this to happen immediately after birth has a long list of benefits! So, barring special circumstances, this is a fantastic way to welcome your baby into the world.

Skin-to-skin contact with your baby stimulates oxytocin, another amazing design feature of the birthing process. It turbocharges the bonding process, helping you to want to protect and nurture your baby immediately. However, it is important to say, even with the oodles of oxytocin coursing around their veins, some people take a little while to connect with their baby fully, and if this is you, that's OK and a normal response, too.

As we said above, the oxytocin not only helps with attachment bonding, but it also begins stimulating the uterus, so that within the hour you'll have birthed your placenta.

When your baby lies directly on your bare chest – and on your partner's, too – they start to colonize with your friendly bacteria, which is amazing because it means alongside the antibodies in your milk (if you're choosing to breastfeed or chestfeed), you begin protecting your little one from any unsavoury bugs and germs that may be lurking.

One of the by-products of oxytocin production is a warm, fuzzy feeling. The warmth helps to start regulating baby's body temperature and reduces their cortisol levels (the stress hormone). It also triggers your milk ducts so that you can begin feeding baby right away.

If, due to special circumstances, you're unable to move forward with immediate skin to skin, but it's something you don't want to miss out on – particularly if your baby is preterm – you can always ask your care providers about Kangaroo Care. This is where you get to carry baby around on your chest, like a little joey, which again helps to form attachment, helps with breastfeeding/chestfeeding and importantly, colonizes baby with your friendly bacteria to help protect against illness and infection. Ultimately, it is NEVER too late to initiate skin to skin and keep it going for as long as you like!

Breastfeeding/chestfeeding/feeding

We don't assume to know how you intend to feed your baby. Whether you choose to breastfeed or formula feed is entirely up to you. It is important that, as with birth, you dispel any misconceptions or fears you have about breastfeeding, understand the pros and cons of all feeding options available to you and make an informed choice – one that is right for you and your family. It is important to do this in the antenatal period so that when your baby is born, you're clear on how you want to feed and feel confident with your choice. Breastfeeding or chestfeeding, as with birth, is an individual journey that for some people comes very naturally, and for others can be extremely challenging – hence the suggestion to prepare during your pregnancy.

Western society has conditioned us to sexualize our breasts. Many clients have told us that they choose not to breastfeed because they feel uncomfortable at the thought or they worry about the impact it will have on their sex life. Some of you may read that and think it is a ridiculous reason not to breastfeed but just look at how the media objectifies and portrays breasts! By unpicking worries and thoughts like this (the primary function of your breasts is to feed your offspring and there is absolutely no reason why breastfeeding would impact your sex life) you can begin to see the beauty (and health benefits) that lie within a breastfeeding journey.

While we don't go into any details about the practicalities in this book, please do check out our amazing two-for-one offer which includes The Calm Birth School online video course and The Mindful Breastfeeding course (featuring founder Anna Le Grange) at www.thecalmbirthschool.com/ the-calm-birth-school-and-the-mindful-breastfeeding-2-for-1-bundle/ and the audio provided as part of our book bonuses.

It is a good idea to initiate breastfeeding within the first hour of birth (the golden hour). Just as skin to skin helps to produce oxytocin and encourages the release of the placenta, so does the action of your baby feeding at your chest. You can ask for support from your care providers too if you feel you need guidance in helping baby to latch on (although please be aware that not all midwives or healthcare professionals are experts in breastfeeding). Alternatively, you could research 'the breastcrawl', which occurs when a newborn baby is placed on their birth parent's chest or abdomen immediately after birth and (given the time to do so) will naturally begin rooting and using their newborn reflexes to find the parent's nipple and begin to feed without the support of parent or health professional latching them on! It is amazing. Aside from the obvious benefits of skin to skin, it is thought that the breastcrawl creates a better latch and improves early feeding outcomes.

We will talk more about the emotional side of breastfeeding in the next chapter, but for now a note on formula feeding. Please know that you aren't any less a loving parent if you choose (or switch) to formula. You haven't failed your child. Trust that you have made a choice that, at the time, was right for you and your family.

CHAPTER 21

What Happens Now?

So, let's put those visualization skills to work now and imagine you navigated pregnancy, you prepped like a badass and you birthed like one too. (No matter how that came to fruition, you gave birth and you're amazing. End. Of.) What happens now?

It sometimes feels like an unwritten rule that we don't tell people what the postnatal period can really be like – almost like a fight club rule: *What happens in the fourth trimester, stays in the fourth trimester* – but we can learn so much from each other (without scaring the be-jaysus out of each other). So, I'm going to tell you... the truth – the truth about that bit that comes after the birth of your baby.

It can be wonderful and it can be bloody hard.

Once your baby is born, you expect to feel so appreciative of all that you now have. You expect to feel happy and connected to your baby, that your instincts are razor-sharp and that you know exactly what to do. You expect to feel like your life is complete. You might feel like that and if you do, that is wonderful – truly wonderful. But you might also feel like you have no idea how to look after a baby; you might not feel the instant love that everyone talks about. You might feel like it is really hard work and that you don't know whose opinion to listen to. You might even think you have made a mistake!

Perhaps it will be a mixture of all these. Maybe you'll feel one way one day and totally different the next. Either way, it's all normal and all OK (we will talk about what might not be OK a little later on). None of this defines who you are as a parent, how 'good' a parent you are or how happy your child will be. None of it.

I (Liz), remember clearly after having my first child, that I had focused so much on the pregnancy, reducing my fear and preparing for birth (which was all needed) that I hadn't even considered what it would be like to be a parent to a tiny human who needed my constant touch, love and support just to stay alive! That is a scary thought, right? Well, when it dawned on me, within hours of her being born, it terrified me.

My only reference to what the 'new baby' period was like was my sister's experience. She'd had her child nine months before me and she pretty much breezed it (proof that you CAN experience it that way!). But I'm not my sister, and reflectively, I know I would have benefited from some antenatal preparation for breastfeeding, some kind of postnatal preference planning session and recognition that my hypnobirthing tools could support me through this new, unnavigated and challenging period in my life. You know yourself better than anyone. What do you need to do to prepare for this life-altering, all-consuming yet AMAZING time in your life?

The postnatal period is, in my opinion, one of the most life-changing periods that could occur in a person's life. Yes, you might breeze through it, and I hope you do – but you're more likely to have a positive postnatal period if you put some planning and thought into it (I know, I know, more to think about!).

Let's get into the nuts and bolts of the fourth trimester: what you need to consider and how you can shape it to be more magical than daunting.

The most important thing in the postnatal period is…**YOU**!

You're your baby's everything. Their safety and security, their love, their warmth, their sustenance and their support system. This was effortless (almost!) for you to provide while you were pregnant, but as baby transitions earthside and you step into your role as a parent those things that your baby wants, needs and expects can be exhausting to provide. This is why it is so, so, *so* important that you're taking care of yourself. Don't just read that and think 'yeah, yeah' or skip to the next bit – get this part nailed and the rest will feel so much easier. Keep that in mind as you care for your child and parenting will feel less daunting.

Making yourself a priority could be as simple as having conversations with those around you now. Consider questions like:

- What role will my partner play in the postnatal period? If you don't have this conversation before baby is born, you might find that you both have totally different expectations.

- Who will support all of us? This could be your mum, sister, other family member, a BFF or a postnatal doula (*see pages 255–258 to find recommendations*).

- How will we manage to feed ourselves healthy meals? Consider asking friends and family to make you a meal you can pop in the freezer and easily heat up when you need it.

- How will we get enough sleep? If you're up feeding in the night, will your partner (or someone else) be able to take care of the baby for an hour (or two) during the day, so you can catch up on sleep?

- Who will do the chores? Be prepared to have to let go of some of the household chores and not be Mary Poppins, but discuss with your partner about what they will need to be responsible for in the early days of the postnatal period. What are the things that you really can't let slide?

- How will I take care of my other children (if you have any)? Discuss any childcare options and logistics to give you peace of mind.

Once you have had an open conversation like this you begin to create the foundations for a positive postnatal period. Simple things, like having support in place and feeling supported, eating well, getting 'some' sleep, really do go far!

Feeding your baby

As we mentioned in the previous chapter, you might choose to breastfeed, you might not. If you're undecided, use BRAINS to help you make a decision. It is your choice, and no one should be allowed to make you feel negative about how you choose to feed your baby.

What we would like to touch upon is the emotional side of feeding because, next to the lack of sleep, it's often one of the things that most takes new parents by surprise. Ensuring your child has enough nourishment is solely down to you if you choose to breastfeed. If you find that everything does not fall into place naturally around breastfeeding, the feelings of guilt and shame at not being able to feed your baby in the way you had envisaged can be overwhelming.

The evidence shows that statistically, those who seek out support and guidance before their baby arrives tend to have a more positive breastfeeding/chestfeeding experience. Those who look for assistance from a lactation consultant as early as possible if things aren't going as well as anticipated are far more likely to breastfeed/chestfeed for longer. Don't suffer in silence or wait for six weeks before acknowledging that help would be good. Needing help does not make you a failure.

If, after seeking out support, you still feel as though breastfeeding isn't for you, please do not beat yourself up. The happiest children have happy mothers and caregivers. Sometimes, for a multitude of reasons, you may choose to stop breastfeeding/chestfeeding. Please hear that this doesn't make you a bad person or a bad mother. Educate and empower yourself, and remember it's your body, your baby, your decision and nobody else's business.

Although I really recommend you doing some antenatal prep for breastfeeding/chestfeeding, (see *The Mindful Breastfeeding School*)[57] you can use your hypnobirthing techniques to support you through your feeding journey, too. In fact, the tips below apply whatever your mode of feeding is:

- Each time you feed your baby is an opportunity to connect with them. Hard to do when you might be feeling harassed, tired or anxious, but counteract those feelings by holding your baby close (skin to skin where possible) and adopt your Calm Birth School Breathing. This will help you to relax, release oxytocin and be in the moment.

- Listen to our New Mama/New Parent affirmations when you feed and repeat the phrases to help you build up your confidence in your parenting and boost your feel-good hormones.

Anna Le Grange, from The Mindful Breastfeeding School, has provided a breastfeeding audio to help you to relax while you feed your baby.

Sleep

Ah sleep... elusive sleep. For some time after having a baby, sleep will likely be a hot topic of conversation for you! In our experience, having realistic expectations of how a newborn sleeps will help you adjust to your new (sleep-deprived!) normal. Babies do not sleep like adults – trust me (Liz), this was a huge shock to me with my first baby!

A baby's sleep cycle is around 45 minutes (compared to an adult's which is 90 minutes); sometimes they may transition back into sleep after a cycle and sometimes they might wake. A baby has 12–16 sleep cycles per night which yes, means they could wake 16 times in one night. According to Sarah Oakwell-Smith (author of *The Gentle Sleep Book*,[58] which we recommend you read) this is actually a good thing! Although it may be exhausting for parents, the frequent waking keeps your baby safe and protects them against SIDS.[59] You may also want to consider the benefits of safe co-sleeping with your baby, which can make it easier for you to respond to them, enable them to settle more quickly and hopefully allow you to get some better-quality sleep, too.

Now you know that some sleep deprivation is pretty inevitable, and that it happens for a reason, it may feel easier to accept that this is your short-term reality. While you transition into this period, here are a few tips to help you feel as energized as possible:

- When you wake for the day (for what might feel like the hundredth time!) energize your body by using your hypnobirthing breathing skills. Take three deep, slow breaths into your abdomen, filling your lungs up and matching the length of your breath in and out. If you have a caesarean birth scar, be careful not to push your stomach out too far; go with what feels good to you.

- Visualize yourself standing tall and strong in nature, your feet grounded to the earth. I won't ask you to hug any trees (although you really should try it!) but you could go as far as noticing that there are roots growing from under the soles of your feet rooting you to the earth and helping you to stand strong. Take another couple of deep breaths as you do this.

- Repeat an affirmation or a mantra in your mind a few times. You could create one yourself or try: 'The more I relax, the easier things feel', 'I remember to trust my inner wisdom' or 'I am a calm and confident mother/parent.'

- Listen to a 20-minute meditation track during the day. We have all heard the saying 'sleep when baby sleeps', which isn't always possible, but taking 20 minutes to meditate can have similar benefits to taking a nap and help you to navigate the rest of your day/evening more easily.

Emotions

Oh boy… emotions after having a baby are can be All.The. Things. Known as 'the baby blues', they can leave you blissfully happy one minute and desperately sad the next. In this time, it is important to lean into the emotions, feel what you're feeling and accept that this is a part of the 'newborn' phase. For most people this is short-lived and feelings and emotions begin to settle after 10–14 days. Things that may help are:

- talking with your partner or a trusted friend about how you're feeling

- listening to your New Mama/Parent affirmations

- doing your TCBS breathing (in for four and out for seven)

- getting as much sleep or rest as possible.

The baby blues are normal and are experienced by most. It is the impact of the hormone changes in your body, and your body and mind adjusting to not being pregnant any more. Sometimes after giving birth, people experience feelings of hopelessness, sadness, guilt or self-blame – if this lasts for more than a few weeks, it could be postnatal depression (PND). One in 10 mothers/birthing parents will experience this to varying different degrees. Unlike the baby blues, PND is a mental health condition that requires support, which might be in the form of a talking therapy, medication, self-help or perhaps all three. Please note that some people can experience a similar condition during pregnancy known as 'prenatal depression'. Hypnobirthing can still be part of your preparation for birth if you experience this, but it is important to seek support (or treatment) from your GP, midwife or healthcare professionals as well.

Anxiety is also a common mental health condition to experience during pregnancy or in the postnatal period. It can sometimes be a symptom of PND or can be experienced on its own. Utilizing the hypnobirthing techniques you used during pregnancy can help to manage the symptoms of anxiety, but it is always best to get advice from a mental health professional or your doctor.

There are other mental health conditions to be aware of that affect a smaller number of people after giving birth such as postpartum psychosis, obsessive compulsive disorder (OCD) and post-traumatic stress disorder (PTSD).

If you experience any mental health conditions during pregnancy or after giving birth, then please seek support and know that you're not weak, a bad parent or 'just not cut out for this' and most importantly, you can get better. As someone who has experienced perinatal mental health issues [Liz has had depression, anxiety and OCD], I know that a full recovery is absolutely possible.

Physical healing

Whether you have the most gentle, calm birth ever, you require some assistance to birth your baby or you have an abdominal birth, chances are that your body will need to heal.

Here are some ideas for you to take note of and explore:

- The most important thing here is time. Give yourself TIME to heal. There is no need to be a superhero. There is nothing to prove. You don't need to be out and about immediately. Take things easy for at the least the first few weeks of the postnatal period (if not the first month) and you'll reap the benefits of it later.

- Consider a 'closing the bones' ceremony, which involves the use of a traditional shawl called a 'rebozo', to rock and move the mother's hips, followed by an abdominal and pelvic massage, and finished by tightly wrapping the cloth around your hips. This process helps to release emotions and stimulates blood flow which, in turn, helps to balance hormones and bolster the immune system.

- Take a look at belly binding – this involves wrapping a material (like a rebozo) around your abdomen. The material is usually wrapped tightly and helps to provide support and keep your abdomen in place. This can be helpful, as your body will continue to experience changes after giving birth, and that support it offers can help your body heal properly.

Why not think ahead now and book in a treatment like the above for the postnatal period?

Relationships

Inevitably, relationships change, evolve and grow in the postnatal period. Having open, direct, compassionate communication with your partner and loved ones will help to ensure that the evolution is a positive one.

A common concern for some people is visitors after birth. Often, we can feel compelled to 'entertain' friends and family and parade our baby about, passing them from one family member to another. Of course, it is lovely to introduce your little one to their extended circle of important people, but it can feel *too much* in this very new, vulnerable period of your life. If you're worried about this, consider speaking to your partner now about it, and decide how you'll handle any requests to meet baby in the very early days. Don't be afraid to say no – this is a very special time for your new family and the more time you have to connect with your new normal (with trusted support people in place), the better!

When you feel ready, having a community you can turn to or lean on during the postnatal period is vital. Building up connections during pregnancy with other parents-to-be and being open with those you already have around you is pivotal in helping you to have a positive postnatal experience.

The most amazing relationship started at the conception of your baby (as we discussed in Chapter 9). You can nurture that relationship and bond with your baby at any time during pregnancy and reap the benefits of that in the postnatal period. Now, during this time, connect with your baby in whichever way feels most natural to you: for example, when you're connecting with your baby *physically*, practise skin to skin as often as possible, talk to your baby, make eye contact with them and make space for that love to grow, and to grow between you. Your partner can get involved too by doing the same thing. Just stare in wonder at the amazing miracle you have created and feel all those feelings! It is so magical!

Parenting... it literally lasts for ever!

The best piece of advice I had when I had two small children and was struggling to understand how everyone else was managing to make it look effortless and I wasn't, came from my cousin, who told me, 'Liz, kids are as hard work as you make them.' I can't tell you how much this little nugget changed my approach. I realized that I was trying to get my babies to fit into the ideals that were being reflected to me by social media, television, etc. and not tuning in to them as little individuals. I was judging myself based on an external standard that shouldn't apply to me or anyone else. I was making them feel like hard work by expecting them to be a certain way.

Beyond the immediate postnatal period, if you feel you want to explore a similar approach to hypnobirthing, but for parenting, I would highly recommend you explore hypnoparenting, a hypnosis-based programme for parents, helping them take back control, reduce overwhelm and find more joy in their lives. The programme was founded and created by Jade Gordon, who has very kindly provided a lovely bonus video to tell you how you can take all the useful techniques you learned in hynpobirthing and integrate them to help you approach parenthood in a calmer way.

It might feel like there is so much to navigate during pregnancy, birth and in the postnatal period, but with some preparation and tuning in to and trusting your own instincts, you can make this somewhat uncertain and vulnerable time in your life a truly positive, transformative experience.

Conclusion: Moving Forward

I hope as you reach the end of this book a quiet confidence has been awakened within you, or that perhaps the inner strength that you have been silently drawing upon now has its own voice, which you feel very comfortable sharing with the world.

Hypnobirthing isn't about producing perfect 'textbook' births. If only it were that easy. However, when as a birthing woman or person you understand what you can control, and you let go of what you can't, you can step into creating the most positive birth experience, regardless of the way your baby chooses to enter into the world.

This is your body, your baby and your unique experience. You're a warrior, a marvellous creation who was born to give birth. You now know that birth is a natural and normal event, not a medical condition.

You know that being able to embrace and accept what is going on in your body, rather than resist it, can help you to manage the sensations of birth far more effectively.

You understand that, although your emotional state will have a huge impact on the way that you experience birth, the birth environment, your care providers and your birth partner also have extremely important roles, and all of them should be there to support you fully. You have the right to ask for what you want and need.

You now have a toolkit of specific techniques that will help you to remain feeling calm and at ease throughout your labour and birth (and into the postnatal period too).

So what's next?

No one can force you to do anything you don't want to do, but in order to get the most out of this book, we suggest that you go right back to the beginning and read it again, highlighting all the salient points. Yes, seriously. Remember everything we've said about preparation. Never underestimate its value.

There really is no secret to giving birth, other than to be present in any given moment and to accept what is going on with your body. The nub is, for most of us out there, that it takes time and practice to be able to tap into the acceptance that you need on the day. So hear me when I say that I believe in you and you've got this – and make sure you put the time in, do your practice and watch how you're able to take whatever birth sends your way with ease.

Next, set dedicated time aside in your calendar to practise the breathing techniques and visualizations. Don't simply set the intention to practise: by putting actual appointments into your calendar, you'll make the appointments with yourself 'real' and will be much more likely to show up for them – especially if you've got a full life already. Remember to visit www.thecalmbirthschool.com/bookbonuses where you can download The Calm Birth Method practice guide.

In closing, I want you to know, it's so not about birth for me, it's about life. This is about *you*. I want you to know that you count and your voice is important.

Giving birth should never define a person. Yet the process of fully connecting with your inner voice, strength and wisdom as you learn to exercise, stretch, pull and embody, during both your pregnancy and birth, will provide you with an opportunity to celebrate and own your magnificence. Not only as a human being who is a living, breathing, walking miracle, but also as someone who creates miracles.

As you gain confidence in communicating your needs, wishes and desires for you and your unborn baby you begin to understand the power that you contain is the power needed to conquer worlds, whether these worlds are within the private sanctuary of your home, or breaking down glass ceilings in the boardroom. This path (while not the only way) is a path to your power in life.

It starts with knowing what you want and telling other people, then looking your fear in the face. Staring at it head-on and seeing it melt away as you trust in yourself, your body and your baby and lean into your strength.

When you can navigate your birth in a way that leaves you feeling like a warrior. It changes things.

It changes you.

You know you can do anything. You can do ANYTHING.

You've got this!

All the love

Suzy and Liz xo

Postscript

More birth stories? Oh, go on then!

❧ Hayley's birth story ❧

Today is my due date. However, six days ago our little Huxley Isaac decided to come into the world.

My waters released at 11:30 p.m. on Sunday. I called the midwife and she suggested going back to bed as it could be a while before anything happened. (I'd been having really strong Braxton Hicks for a week.) I managed to doze off until about 4:30 a.m. then decided to get up; the surges were mild and 10 minutes apart, so I called my mum at 5:30 a.m. to come over to help get our four-year-old to school.

I then spent the next few hours trying to doze off, walking around the house and having small snacks, all the while welcoming the surges. I found walking and standing up for them was the only way to cope with them. We had lavender burning, candles and 'plinky-plonk music' as my other half calls it! It was super relaxing; my mum said she felt as though she was in a spa!

I walked to the end of the garden and back again a few time and the surges (when we timed them, which wasn't all the time) ranged from four minutes to eight or nine minutes apart.

We called the midwives again at 11:30 a.m. They told me to just relax, not do anything, let my body do its thing and, if I wanted, to have a bath. I had a bit of an ache down below but not a pushing feeling, so one midwife advised me to examine myself in the bath to see if I could feel anything. After getting into the bath and feeling what I thought might have been the head, I had three close, strong surges. Luckily, the midwives were already en route.

The next couple of hours went so fast. I had the affirmations on while I rocked, holding on to my partner or my mum, I found 'ahhh-ing' sometimes on the out-breath of wave breathing helped. The pool was only just filled in time; I got in at 3:18 p.m. and only three surges later at 3:34 p.m. our baby boy arrived!

I am so thrilled with our calm, positive birth experience, which, despite being definitely uncomfortable at times towards the end, was also in a way euphoric. This birth was 16 hours from start to finish compared with 30 hours with my first. I only had three surges where I let go and birthed him compared with two and half hours of forced pushing with my first. We were in the comfort of our home and tucked up in bed within an hour!

Thank you to The Calm Birth School for everything I've learned, for changing my perception of birth – as well my mum's and hopefully others' too – and all the support I've received from the Facebook group.

๛ Suzy's final birth story – welcoming ๛ Aluna Grace Ashworth into the world

My body tends to like my babies well done. Caesar was born 11 days after my guess date, Coco was born 13 days after hers and after what felt like an exceedingly long wait, Aluna was finally born at home, in the water, delivered, by me – 15 days after her guess date. And it was everything I could have hoped for.

The day before I went into labour started really positively. I visited a new reflexologist and, I'm not going to lie, there was part of me that was hoping the treatment was going to shimmy things along. But as I say frequently during The Calm Birth School video course: 'Natural methods of induction are only useful if baby is on the verge of coming. If baby is not, nothing's going to work.'

Later that day my lovely midwife Virginia Howes came to see me. A couple of days before, I had told her if nothing had happened by Monday, I wanted to have a sweep. So when Virginia arrived she checked for baby's heartbeat and then asked if I still wanted a sweep. When I said yes, being pretty no-nonsense – which I'd loved right throughout my care – Virginia told me what a 'good' sweep would involve and it didn't sound nice. I'd had sweeps with both of my previous pregnancies and, while they were slightly uncomfortable (and ineffective at kick-starting labour), I'd gone with them as the lesser evil over potentially having to have an induction. With this pregnancy, I'd opted to have an independent midwife and so the only conversations I'd had about induction were with other mums at the school gates.

Virginia, and Lauren Durret, my doulas from The Whole Nine Months, were completely supportive and clear that induction was not on the agenda for me. The baby had been crazily active throughout my pregnancy and, while she was still moving around like a mad thing and my blood pressure was as it should be, there didn't seem to be any reason why I should go in for an induction – and particularly with my past history of carrying late.

However, I was now on day 14 past my guess date and, although I felt great after my reflexology, there was part of me that felt I'd done pretty well in terms of staying calm and mostly positive, and if I wanted a sweep I wasn't letting myself or anyone down. Despite that, the thought of Virginia rooting around my nether regions for five minutes trying to stimulate my uterus wasn't appealing, and so before we went down that avenue I asked for a vaginal examination (the only VE I had during my entire pregnancy and birth).

It was uncomfortable, and when Virginia reported back she didn't give me the feedback I wanted to hear. I knew it wouldn't stay that way and I remembered my own advice about it only being a 'moment in time', but it still took a while to get my head round the idea that it wasn't my time yet.

I messaged Lauren to let her know, and she immediately sent back some reassuring words – even though I didn't appreciate them at the time. But that's the beauty of having a doula – you don't have to reassure them, they are there for you and your feelings 100 per cent. Anyway, I decided to hunker down, on went Netflix and I watched films back to back until about 11 p.m. when I switched on Billions. Not the type of programme you watch when you're looking for an oxytocin fix, but what the heck, I wasn't going to go into labour that night anyway. During Billions, the baby started going crazy; my belly was like her own personal punchbag, it was really full-on and about 15 minutes before it ended I noticed that I was feeling quite damp. I'd been losing quite a lot of discharge (apologies if that's TMI) and so I didn't really think too much of it. Then I could feel myself losing more water and thought, Hang on a minute. *I stood up and there was a wet patch on the sofa. Woohoo!! My waters had released (I have a leather sofa, so no damage was done).*

I was super excited, because my waters hadn't released outside active labour before, so I really wasn't expecting it. Of course, as soon as I stood up, there was no question about what was happening. It wasn't a big gush but enough to make me hop, half-run (really, in my condition) to the bathroom, so I could sit on the loo, check that the waters were clear and grab a towel. By this time it was midnight. I was so excited! It did cross my mind that I was already pretty tired; I should have been in bed by 10 p.m. and I wondered if things really were going to kick off that night. As I got into bed, my husband opened one eye and I told him my waters had released and he looked like he might get up for about half a second, before I said it was fine, and, of course, half a second later he was completely asleep again – #men.

As I relaxed in bed the first thing I reached for was my phone. I messaged Virginia and Lauren to let them know the good news and then on went the audio downloads. First I put on the birth rehearsal, which had had me feeling super emotional in the lead-up to birth, and then the fear release... It was important that I listened to that, as even though I was ready, there had been lots of points in the pregnancy where I had questioned whether I was doing enough practice and also felt the pressure of needing to have a great birth. I wanted to let those concerns go, so I could just concentrate on the job in hand. I was hoping that I might be able to go to sleep, but what I had thought were pre-labour surges (and in fact, were actual surges) were too intense to sleep through.

So I just listened to the audio downloads, sat up slightly in bed and focused on my breathing. I did this until just before 3 a.m., when I thought I would try and lie down on my side... immediately everything felt super intense and I realized I needed the toilet. Again, I was really pleased I needed to do a poo and it was pretty loose (I'm doing it again aren't I? TMI!), so I decided to get the hubby up and ask him to fill the pool. Jerome got up straight away and I got busy messaging Virginia and Lauren.

I'd been timing my surges for a while and I was experiencing three surges in 10 minutes, ranging anything from 40–60 seconds. So when Virginia asked me if I wanted her to come, I hesitated before getting back to her, because I didn't want her to come out at 3 a.m. if she didn't have to. But given she was an hour's drive away, I thought it would probably be best if she did make her way over, because who knew what would be happening at 4 a.m., and I was pretty quick with Coco. I then messaged Lauren and took up my position in the living room. I had my laptop by my side, which was playing a slide show of the family photoshoot that the lovely Philippa James had taken a few weeks before, and the TCBS audio playlist was on a loop. I had chosen the Powerball and the Birth Rehearsal affirmations to listen to throughout the birth. Instinctively, I sat down on my knees, facing the sofa with my arms resting on the seat, supporting my head. I had stopped timing by this stage and whenever I felt a surge I circled my hips. Everything felt really manageable. I couldn't have told you how far along I was but I felt very calm, in control. If I had to guess, I would have thought I was still quite early on.

On reflection, time passed really quickly, because before I knew it Virginia was there by my side watching me wind my hips around a surge. She asked me if my surges were any more intense, but I couldn't give an honest answer, because I didn't know. I just knew that it was all quite manageable. As the surge passed, I think Virginia had a listen to baby and all was well. I hung out for a short time longer in the dark of the living room before moving into the kitchen, which was all set beautifully for me by Jerome. There were candles running along the counter tops, our fairy-light wreath hanging by the door, affirmations pinned up along the window and the wall. It was perfect. And when I moved into the kitchen, he brought the laptop so I could continue listening to the playlist on low.

Even though the pool was prepared, I wasn't quite ready to get in. So I resumed the position I had been in, in the living room on my knees, this time leaning on the seat of a chair. I think Virginia must have sensed things were moving along, as she asked me if I was ready to get into the pool. I think I said no to start with and then a little time later she reminded me I could get into the pool if I wanted. I remember feeling that I might as well, but as soon as I did, I simultaneously felt amazing about getting into the water, but also more aware of the surges. The frequency of the surges immediately increased and I had to bring all my awareness to reciting my affirmations. I smile when I think about what I was reciting to myself on the day. The one that sticks out was, 'I am a goddess.' I also said many times, 'I can do this.' And I had to remind myself to release all the tension from my body.

I remember leaning over the pool (same position on my knees leaning forward over the edge) and being aware that it was getting lighter and looking out over the garden and thinking how beautiful it looked. Then feeling like I needed to go for a wee. I told Virginia that I wanted to get out to go to the loo. My surges were coming thick and fast at this point and she told me I could go in the pool, but I wasn't up for that. It's really interesting that I was completely present in between my surges this time, which was very different to Coco's birth, where I stayed 'in the zone' throughout.

Jerome had been quietly watching and supporting from the side of the pool at this point and Virginia asked him to help me out before the next surge arrived. Too late – the next one came! I just managed to get out of the pool when the next one came and it was really intense. Maybe partly because I had got out of the water, but also because I didn't really need a wee... which totally threw both Virginia and me! I talk about baby pressing on the bladder, which can cause some women to go for a poo during labour or to at least feel like they want to go for a poo. When this happened to me this time, because I felt as though I wanted to go for a wee, I didn't realize that it was the baby moving down past my bladder and neither did Virginia. She later said that in all her time of midwifery, no one had ever said they wanted to go for a wee and been at that stage before. So, out of the pool I was standing and as I said I experienced this most intense surge, I lost a lot of water and I pooped! Yep, just a little one but out it came, as my body's natural expulsive reflex kicked into play.

It feels weird to write this here, but this stage totally took me by surprise and my body tensed, I felt another really strong surge and the baby's head began to emerge. I was stuck. I didn't quite know what to do at this point. Virginia told me to get back in the pool; I didn't want to move, but she calmly told me to get back in before the next surge and Jerome helped me back into the water. I put my hand around the back of me and could feel the top of Aluna's head, although I didn't tell Virginia or Jerome I could feel it. I could feel all of the hair. I was still in a bit of shock. I remember feeling the tension in my body and I said to Jerome 'it hurts' and I knew I had to surrender, so I finally made the decision to allow my body to sink into the water.

As I did this, the next surge took over and Aluna's whole head was out. The hardest part was over.

I brought my left hand down between my legs and, as I surged again, guided Aluna out, and Virginia then guided her around to the front. Again, I think I was a bit shell-shocked as I didn't immediately pick her up out of the water, which is fine as newborns don't breathe in until the cold air hits their face. After what probably wasn't longer than a couple of seconds, I lifted her to my chest and then came a rush of emotion that felt so different to my previous two births: the joy and relief that the oxytocin had done it. I had just had a quick, intense, powerful, beautiful birth and delivered my own baby and there she was, full head of hair, beautiful brown eyes, just lying on my chest; it was amazing.

As always the toughest part of all my labours was delivering the placenta. Even though Aluna's birth had been super quick – Virginia had arrived at 4 a.m. and we welcomed Aluna by 5 a.m. – it felt as though it had sapped every bit of energy and strength from me and I made more of a fuss delivering the placenta than I had the baby! Go figure!

Lauren had arrived and was telling me to use my breathing and I remember thinking I can't breathe! But I did (of course) and the placenta came out and my job was done.

All that was left was for Aluna to start feeding and for me to get my lips around a lovely placenta smoothie. It wasn't until we had been out of the pool for at least 15–20 minutes that I even asked what sex 'it' was. Again I was super shocked, as right throughout my pregnancy everyone had been telling me we were going to have a boy, so I thought we were having a boy. It was amazing to have such a lovely surprise. Coco and Caesar woke up just as Aluna started feeding and came downstairs, eyes wide, not quite believing what they were seeing. It was magical.

We didn't name Aluna until later on that day; it was a toss-up between Luella and Aluna, but as Aluna was born on a full moon, and the name means 'Goddess of the Moon', it seemed very fitting.

I felt and feel so blessed to be able to share this totally magical experience with you. Birth is amazing and I look forward to helping many, many more women through The Calm Birth School Instructors across the UK and through the video course enjoy calm and positive births.

❧ **Liz's third birth story** ❧

On 31 January 2015 (my due date!), my family and I decided to have a lazy day at home; however, in the afternoon we ventured out to a local garden centre. After wondering around and taking part in a wildlife hunt, my waters released (embarrassing!) and we all rushed home so I could get some dry clothes. My daughter was super excited, and my little boy was very confused and more concerned about his balloon, which had floated away in the excitement!

Once at home, I relaxed with my family and the surges started over the next few hours. I had been painstakingly planning a home birth with a birthing pool. My birthing room had positive affirmations, poems from my Mother's Blessing and pictures drawn by my children adorning it. I created a relaxing environment with candles and my aromatherapy oils, sat on my birthing ball and just enjoyed how things were unfolding. The midwife popped in to see me and then left me to it. My son and daughter were my oxytocin and endorphins: they were so funny and sweet. I was laughing through lots of surges because of them! My mum came round and the kids went to bed and were very well behaved.

The surges started to get closer together, longer and stronger, so my husband, Mike, got the pool ready. Little did I know that there was a problem with our hot water and he ended up boiling water in every pot and pan in the house while my mum and I relaxed and breathed through the surges upstairs. But then... things started to go backwards! My surges were getting further apart and not lasting as long... and stayed like that! The pool was getting colder, so at this point we decided to call the midwife. She came and examined me and I was 3cm dilated. At that point I knew I wasn't progressing, so it wasn't a surprise and I knew I could continue for as long as needed with my hypnobirthing techniques.

The midwife told me I had a temperature, which was a concern because my waters had been gone for quite a while and the longer my labour continued, the higher the chances of infection. The midwife went and left us to it for a couple of hours. She came back a few times and my temperature hadn't gone down. On the third occasion she came to see me with a supervisor of midwives and I was advised to transfer to hospital. My temperature was now accompanied by chills and fever, so I knew that the risk of infection was greater. I knew it was my decision and I was still in control, so I agreed to the transfer. It felt like the right thing. After some tears and a 15-minute wobble because it wasn't what I had planned or wanted, we set off to the hospital. I knew there was a high possibility that I would have to have continuous monitoring of baby, intravenous *antibiotics for me and a possible speeding up of labour with a Syntocinon drip. All of which would restrict my movement and make my labour more challenging.*

I decided in the car that I was going to get in the right frame of mind. I practised self-hypnosis all the way, and visualized my temperature decreasing, over and over again. I know the power of the mind, so I focused all my attention on visualizing my temperature reducing because that was the thing causing all my problems.

I arrived at the nearest hospital that would cater for my now high-risk birth and as soon as I stepped out into the car park I experienced a strong surge and had to lean on Mike while I breathed through it. When we were shown into our room, Mike straight away tried to make me feel more comfortable by putting out a picture of our children and making the room seem more familiar. Our midwife came and introduced herself. At first, I was worried she would be quite dictatorial, due to my new circumstances – but she was excellent. When she examined me she discovered, lo and behold, that my temperature had gone right down! All of that visualization had worked!! There was no need for antibiotics! I had experienced several more strong surges by this point and after a vaginal examination she informed me I was now 8cm dilated! The self-hypnosis had worked a treat! So, my labour was moving much, much quicker – meaning there was no need for intervention or a Syntocinon drip. She made a real effort to read my birthing preferences and to help me to incorporate as much of it as she could into the new situation. My baby was continuously monitored for the rest of my labour, but I told the midwife there was no way I was lying on the bed the whole time! I sat on a chair for a while, stood holding onto Mike and eventually got on my hands and knees on the bed. It meant she had to hold the monitors in place most of the time, but

I zoned out of what she was doing. Looking back, I am so grateful that she did this for me. Mike and my mum were with me all the way, and were fantastic birthing companions. During each surge Mike reminded me to relax my shoulders, my jaw and to breathe. He used an anchor we had practised, which worked brilliantly! Mum kept a cool cloth on my forehead and kept telling me to lean into it while I breathed my baby down. No forced pushing, just instinctual breathing and quite a lot of moo-ing!! The sensations were intense, and I needed my hypnobirthing techniques to support me, but never once did I think, this is painful, and I didn't even consider asking for drugs. Before I knew it, and honestly to my surprise, I felt my baby's head just pop out! No burning, no 'ring of fire'. After the head was out I felt stunned and waited for the next surge so I could meet my baby. When he was fully born, Mike declared, 'It's a boy!' Which was a shock because we had both been convinced we were having a girl!

As per my birth preferences, we waited until the cord stopped pulsating, and I birthed my placenta. I had about two hours of lovely skin to skin with our baby boy and gave him time to crawl instinctively to the breast.

After a shower, I reflected on the fact that, despite the challenges that had arisen, I had given birth to our gorgeous boy, Jamie, drug-free, intervention-free and within two hours of arriving at hospital. All thanks to hypnobirthing! I transferred to the ward and was greeted by my lovely children, who got to cuddle their baby brother. I stayed in overnight for monitoring, but we were both absolutely fine. The kids love Jamie and I am in awe of him!

Endnotes

1. Gas and air is also known as nitrous oxide and by the commercial name, Entonox.

2. Ayers, S. et al. (2006) 'The Effects of Childbirth-Related Post-Traumatic Stress Disorder on Women and Their Relationships: A Qualitative Study', *Psychology, Health & Medicine*, 11(4): 389–98: http://dx.doi.org/10.1080/13548500600708409 [Accessed 15 May 2022].

3. ibid.

4. Beck, C. et al. (2011) 'Posttraumatic Stress Disorder in New Mothers: Results From a Two-Stage U.S. National Survey': https://pubmed.ncbi.nlm.nih.gov/21884230/ [Accessed 15 May 2022].

5. A 'near miss' refers to situations where women nearly died during pregnancy, childbirth or after pregnancy and they survived either by chance or because of the good quality of care they received.

6. Darwin, Z. and Greenfield, M. (2019) 'Mothers and Others: The Invisibility of LGBTQ People in Reproductive and Infant Psychology', *Journal of Reproductive and Infant Psychology*, 37(4): 341–343: www.tandfonline.com/doi/full/10.1080/02646838.2019.1649919 [Accessed 15 May 2022].

7. Greenfield, M. and Darwin, Z. (2021) 'Trans and Non-Binary Pregnancy, Traumatic Birth, and Perinatal Mental Health: A Scoping Review', *International Journal of Transgender Health*, 22(1–2), 203–216, doi: 10.1080/26895269.2020.1841057.

8. Hinds, D. and Hancock, M. (2019) 'One of the Largest Mental Health Trials Launches in Schools': www.gov.uk/government/news/one-of-the-largest-mental-health-trials-launches-in-schools [Accessed 15 May 2022].

9. Matousek, M. (2014) 'The Power of Solitude': www.huffington post.com/mark-matousek/the-power-ofsolitude_b_5276055.html [Accessed 15 May 2022].

10. Zeidan, F. et al. (2012) 'Mindfulness Meditation-Related Pain Relief: Evidence for Unique Brain Mechanisms in the Regulation of Pain', *Neuroscience Letters*, 520(2): 165–73. doi:10.1016/j.neulet.2012.03.082 [Accessed 15 May 2022].

11. Estimated Due Date (EDD). The 'plus' and corresponding number signify the number of days past the EDD the birthing person is. So EDD +8 = eight days past the estimated due date.

12. Condon, J. et al. (2004) 'Surfactant Protein Secreted by the Maturing Mouse Fetal Lung Acts as a Hormone that Signals the Initiation of Parturition', *Proceedings of the National Academy of Sciences*, 101(14): 4978-4983. doi: 10.1073/pnas.0401124101 [Accessed 15 May 2022].

13. Strohbach, V. (2015) *What is the Size of Your Brain?* (Foreword by Dr. Myles Munroe). Bloomington IN: Westbow Press.

14. Also known as a 'membrane sweep' or stretch and sweep, this is a simple procedure in which a care provider will use their fingers to massage the neck of the cervix, in the hope of stimulating the uterus and kick-starting labour.

15. The Foley catheter is a method of induction. It is thin, sterile tubing with an inflatable balloon on one end, which is inserted into the vagina. The balloon is inflated with fluid, causing it to press down on the cervix in order to stimulate it, cause the release of hormones and ripen the cervix.

16. Reitsma A. et al. (2020) 'Maternal Outcomes and Birth Interventions Among Women Who Begin Labour Intending to Give Birth at Home Compared to Women of Low Obstetrical Risk Who Intend to Give Birth in Hospital: A Systematic Review and Meta-Analyses', *EClinicalMedicine*, 21: 100319. doi: 10.1016/j.eclinm.2020.100319

17. Birthrights (2022) 'Choice of Place of Birth': www.birthrights. org.uk/factsheets/choice-of-place-of-birth/ [accessed 22 May 2022].

18. MacDorman, M.F. and Declercq, E. (2019) 'Trends and State Variations in Out-of-Hospital Births in the United States, 2004–2017', *Birth (Berkeley, Calif.)* 46(2): 279–288. doi:10.1111/birt.12411 [Accessed 15 May 2022].

19. Conaway B. (2012) 'How Do You Want to Deliver Your Baby? Find the Childbirth Option That's Right For You': www. webmd.com/baby/features/childbirth-options-whatsbest#3 [accessed 22 May 2022].

20. ibid.

21. Bohren M.A. et al. (2017) 'Continuous Support For Women During Childbirth', *Cochrane Database of Systematic Reviews* 7(7): CD003766. doi: 10.1002/14651858.CD003766.pub6 [accessed 22 May 2022].

22. Bohren M.A. et al (2019) 'Perceptions and Experiences of Labour Companionship: A Qualitative Evidence Synthesis', *Cochrane Database of Systematic Reviews* 3: CD012449, doi: 10.1002/14651858.CD012449.pub2. [accessed 22 May 2022].

23. Labor of Love (2022) 'Sherpa Doula...': https://alaboroflove.org/sherpa-doula/ [Accessed 15 May 2022].

24. MBRRACE-UK (2020) 'Saving Lives, Improving Mothers' Care': www.npeu.ox.ac.uk/assets/downloads/mbrrace-uk/reports/maternal-report-2020/MBRRACE-UK_Maternal_Report_2020_-_Lay_Summary_v10.pdf [Accessed 22 May 2022].

25. NPEU (2020) 'The Birthplace Cohort Study: Key Findings': www.npeu.ox.ac.uk/birthplace/results [Accessed 22 May 2022].

26. GOV.UK (2020) 'Government Working With Midwives, Medical Experts, and Academics to Investigate BAME Maternal Mortality': /www.gov.uk/government/news/government-working-with-midwives-medical-experts-and-academics-to-investigate-bame-maternal-mortality [accessed 22 May 2022].

27. Tikkanen, R. (2020) 'Maternal Mortality and Maternity Care in the United States Compared to 10 Other Developed Countries': www.commonwealthfund.org/publications/

issue-briefs/2020/nov/maternal-mortality-maternity-care-us-compared-10-countries [accessed 22 May 2022].

28. UNFPA (2021) 'The State of the World's Midwifery 2021': www.unfpa.org/sites/default/files/pub-pdf/21-038-UNFPA-SoWMy2021-Report-ENv4302.pdf [accessed 22 May 2022].

29. UNICEF (2019) 'Maternal Mortality': https://data.unicef.org/topic/maternal-health/maternal-mortality/ [accessed 22 May 2022].

30. Tikkanen, R. (2020) 'Maternal Mortality and Maternity Care in the United States Compared to 10 Other Developed Countries': www.commonwealthfund.org/publications/issue-briefs/2020/nov/maternal-mortality-maternity-care-us-compared-10-countries [accessed 22 May 2022].

31. CDC 'Preventing Pregnancy-Related Deaths' (2022) www.cdc.gov/reproductivehealth/maternal-mortality/preventing-pregnancy-related-deaths.html [Accessed 22 May 2022].

32. MBRRACE-UK (2020) 'Saving Lives, Improving Mothers' Care': www.npeu.ox.ac.uk/assets/downloads/mbrrace-uk/reports/maternal-report-2020/MBRRACE-UK_Maternal_Report_2020_-_Lay_Summary_v10.pdf [Accessed 22 May 2022].

33. Note that the updated MBRRACE report (2021) shows that mixed ethnicity women and birthing people's risk has dropped to twice as likely. See: 'Saving Lives, Improving Mothers' Care': www.npeu.ox.ac.uk/assets/downloads/mbrrace-uk/reports/maternal-report-2021/MBRRACE-UK_Maternal_Report_2021_-_Lay_Summary_v10.pdf [Accessed 22 May 2022].

34. House of Commons; House of Lords (2019–21) 'Black People, Racism and Human Rights: Government Response to the Committee's Eleventh Report of Session 2019–21': https://committees.parliament.uk/publications/3376/documents/32359/default/ [Accessed 22 May 2022].

35. Five X More (2022) 'The Black Women's Maternity Experiences Report': www.fivexmore.com/ [Accessed 22 May 2022].

36. Hansard (2019) 'Black Maternal Healthcare and Mortality': https://hansard.parliament.uk/Commons/2021-04-19/

debates/6935B9C7-6419-4E7B-A813-E852A4EE4F5C/
BlackMaternalHealthcareAndMortality [Accessed 22 May 2022].

37. Black Mamas Matter Alliance: https://blackmamas
    matter.org/about/

38. The Royal College of Obstetricians & Gynaecologists (2020)
    'RCOG Position Statement: Racial Disparities in Women's
    Healthcare': www.rcog.org.uk/media/qbtblxrx/racial-
    disparities-womens-healthcare-march-2020.pdf [Accessed
    22 May 2022].

39. Ashworth, E. (2022) 'You Are Allowed to Audio or Video Record
    Your Consultation': www.instagram.com/p/CPXliqQg0SB/
    [Accessed 23 May 2022].

40. Dekker, R. (2019) 'Evidence on: Doulas', Evidence Based Birth®:
    https://evidencebasedbirth.com/the-evidence-for-doulas/
    [Accessed 23 May 2022].

41. Abuela Doulas: https://abueladoulas.co.uk/

42. Prodromal labour is labour that starts and stops before fully
    active labour begins.

43. NSTs (Non Stress Tests) measure baby's heart rate and
    response to movement.

44. The practice of ingesting the placenta after it has been
    steamed, dehydrated, ground and placed into pills.

45. Alfirevic, Z. et al (2013) 'Continuous Cardiotocography
    (CTG) as a Form of Electronic Fetal Monitoring (EFM) for
    Fetal Assessment During Labour', *Cochrane Database of
    Systematic Reviews*, 5: doi: 10.1002/14651858.CD006066.pub2
    [Accessed 17 May 2022].

46. Finucane, E.M. et al. (2020) 'Membrane Sweeping for Induction
    of Labour', *Cochrane Database of Systematic Reviews*,
    2: www.cochranelibrary.com/cdsr/doi/10.1002/14651858.
    CD000451.pub3/full [Accessed 17 May 2022].

47. Hill, M.J. et al. (2008) 'The Effect of Membrane Sweeping on
    Prelabor Rupture of Membranes: A Randomized Controlled
    Trial' *Obstet Gynecol*, 11(6): 1313–9, https://pubmed.ncbi.nlm.
    nih.gov/18515514/ [Accessed 17 May 2022].

48. Positive Induction Birth: Your Guide to a More Positive and Informed Induction Experience (2022): 'Hypnobirthing': https://positiveinduction.com/tag/hypnobirthing/ [Accessed 17 May 2022].

49. Kicks Count (2022) 'Your Baby's Kicks Count': www.kickscount.org.uk/ [Accessed 24 May 2022].

50. Al-Kuran O. et al. (2011) 'The Effect of Late Pregnancy Consumption of Date Fruit on Labour and Delivery', *J Obstet Gynaecol*, 31(1): 29–31, doi: 10.3109/01443615.2010.522267. PMID: 21280989. www.ncbi.nlm.nih.gov/pubmed/21280989 [Accessed 17 May 2022].

51. Reed, R. (2019) 'Pre-Labour Rupture of Membranes: Impatience and Risk': https://midwifethinking.com/2017/01/11/pre-labour-rupture-of-membranes-impatience-and-risk/ [Accessed 22 May 2022]

52. Doppler – an ultrasound test used to detect blood flow using sound waves.

53. Gupta, J.K. et al. (2012) 'Position in the Second Stage of Labour for Women without Epidural Anaesthesia', *Cochrane Database System Review*, 16(5): www.ncbi.nlm.nih.gov/pubmed/22592681 [Accessed 17 May 2022]

54. Horn, A. (2010) 'The Third Stage of Labour: Choosing between Active and Physiological Delivery of the Placenta': www.homebirth.org.uk/thirdstage.htm [Accessed 17 May 2022].

55. The Royal College of Midwives (2022): 'New Labour guidance resource for women': www.rcm.org.uk/news-views/news/2019/new-labour-guidance-resource-for-women/ [Accessed 17 May 2022].

56. Payne, J. (2015) 'Retained Placenta': https://patient.info/doctor/retained-placenta [Accessed 17 May 2022].

57. The Calm Birth School (2022): www.thecalmbirthschool.com/the-calm-birth-school-and-the-mindful-breastfeeding-2-for-1-bundle/ [Accessed 17 May 2022].

58. Ockwell-Smith, S. (2015) *The Gentle Sleep Book*. London: Piatkus.

59. SIDS stands for Sudden Infant Death Syndrome (also known as cot death).

Additional Support and Resources

The Calm Birth School classes

If you would love to have in-person support and find an instructor near you, please visit: www.thecalmbirthschool. com/instructor-directory/ for more information.

The Calm Birth School video programme

While Suzy no longer offers face-to-face classes and Liz offers a very limited number, one way to experience the equivalent of a private class in the comfort and convenience of your own home is to invest in The Calm Birth School video programme. The benefits of this include:

- Being able to control and direct your learning by participating in the classes as many times as you want or need to, right up until the day you go into labour.

- Learning in two different formats – reading and visual/ auditory via the video – which many people find suits their learning style.

- You might find it easier to engage your birth partner in the video programme.

All students of the video programme also get direct access to support through The Calm Birth School closed Facebook group, where you can ask questions, and raise concerns or fears that may come up during your pregnancy journey.

All purchasers of The *Calm Birth Method* can purchase The Calm Birth School course with a 15 per cent discount using the coupon code TCBS15BOOK.

The Calm Birth School training

If you are a birth-passionate person and you want to make your love for supporting people as they prepare for birth your career, join us for a unique and fully comprehensive course providing everything you need to become a professional Hypnobirthing Instructor for The Calm Birth School in under 12 weeks! It is time to change lives and start helping birthing women and people to create the most positive birth experience possible for their own unique situation. Visit www.thecalmbirthschool.com/hypnobirthing-the-instructor-training-programme/ to find out more.

Anti-racism resources

Please visit our padlet (www.padlet.com/liz66/antiracism resources) to take a look at some of TCBS's favourite Anti-Racism resources.

Pregnancy and birth

Birthrights: Promoting dignity and human rights in childbirth: www.birthrights.org.uk

Mama Academy: Empowering mums and midwives to help more babies arrive safely: www.mamaacademy.org.uk

Tell Me A Good Birth Story: Database of 'birth buddies' offering free support to your unique situation: www.tellmeagoodbirthstory.com

BellyBelly Pregnancy and Birth: Pregnancy, birth and parenting website: www.bellybelly.com.au

Birth Trauma Association: If you didn't have the birth you wanted and need some impartial support to help you work through your experience: www.birthtraumaassociation.org.uk

La Leche League GB: Information and encouragement for breastfeeding mothers: www.laleche.org.uk

AIMS: Association for Improvements in the Maternity Services campaigns for better understanding of the normal birth process and provides support and information about maternity choices in the UK and Ireland: www.aims.org.uk

Evidence Based Birth®: Helping you to make empowered, evidence-based decisions about your upcoming birth: https://evidencebasedbirth.com/resources-for-parents/

The Mindful Breastfeeding School: Tools, techniques and lactation support to help parents feed and connect with their baby for a more relaxed, calm and fulfilling early parenting experience: www.mindfulbreastfeeding.co.uk/. Many TCBS Instructors are also trained in Mindful Breastfeeding, which is indicated by a badge next to their directory listing: www.thecalmbirthschool.com/instructor-directory/

Hypnoparenting: Build your mental health resilience with Jade Gordon's course for a calmer, more joyful parenthood without overwhelm, frustration and anxiety: https://courses.sonamum.com/the-hypnoparenting-course

Nurturing Birth: Find the right doula for you, to support you through your pregnancy, birth and postnatal period. Find a doula who is local, respected, informed, supportive and non-judgemental: www.nurturingbirthdirectory.com/

Abuela Doula: Choosing a doula is a very personal thing. Your birthkeeper will walk alongside you as you welcome new life into your home. Your Abuela brings the wisdom of the Abuelas with them: https://abueladoulas.co.uk/

Further reading

Janet Balaskas, *New Active Birth* (Thorsons, 1991)

Dean Beaumont, *The Expectant Dad's Handbook* (Penguin Random House, 2013)

Sarah J. Buckley, *Gentle Birth, Gentle Mothering* (Penguin Random House, 2009)

Sophie Burch, *Beyond Birth; A Mindful Guide to Early Parenting* (self-published, 2021)

Grantly Dick, *Childbirth Without Fear* (Pinter & Martin, 2013)

Eleanor Hayes, *Helping Birth: Your Guide To Pain Relief Choices and interventions in Labour and Childbirth* (Bookzang, 2018)

Sarah Ockwell-Smith, *The Gentle Sleep Book: Gentle, No-Tears, Sleep Solutions for Parents of Newborns to Five-Year-Olds* (Hachette, 2015)

Sophie Messager, *Why Postnatal Recovery Matters* (Pinter & Martin, 2020)

Kicki Hansard, *The Secrets of Birth* (self-published, 2015)

Michel Odent, *Birth Reborn* (Pantheon, 1984)

The Calm Birth School Breathing Techniques at a Glance

The Calm Birth School breathing technique

TCBS breathing is a simple, powerful technique. The reason it is so effective is because it triggers the body's natural calming reflex, which occurs when the out-breath is nearly twice as long as the in-breath (we aim for a count of seven). During your labour, this technique will help you maintain a deep state of calm and you'll use it in between surges. You'll also use it as you feel a surge coming in and once it has subsided.

Ideally, the breath is taken in and out through the nose as opposed to the mouth, as this gives you more control over the flow of air. However, please don't stress if you have a cold when you're birthing. Just breathe through your mouth – it will all be OK.

How to do it

Breathe in deeply to the count of four through the nose, imagining you're filling your lungs right to the bottom. As you breathe out, imagine sending the breath down, so it moves around your baby, down your legs into the tips of your toes and then into the floor. Sometimes, when you're first practising this technique, it's useful to put your hands on either side of your waist, so you can feel the rise and fall as you breathe deeply. It really is as simple as that.

When to do it

Use this technique whenever you find yourself feeling stressed, whether it be at work, with your partner, getting on and off public transport – wherever and whenever. This will help you to relax quickly the more that you practise it. In addition, should you be one of the many women or birthing people who labour quickly, this technique will get you into the birthing zone quickly and easily, once you have become accustomed to using it in your everyday life.

If you're the type of person who takes life in your stride with very little stress, this doesn't make you exempt from practising. It's just as important you carve out some practice time for your Calm Birth School breathing too. Ensure you do one set of Calm Birth School breathing in the morning for five minutes, five minutes at lunchtime and five minutes again in the evening.

Wave breathing

Use wave breathing when you're experiencing a wave or surge.

How to do it

The central idea of wave breathing is to keep both the inhalation and the exhalation even. Breathe in through the nose to the count of seven and out through the mouth for seven.

The role of this breath is to work with the upward motion of the uterus as it rises, and then to send your breath down to your baby and your womb, while relaxing. Simple!

However, don't be fooled. For you to move instinctively into that space of deep breathing and relaxation when you experience a wave, you need to have practised it often so that you're used to it.

Please do not worry if you're unable to keep the breath even for a count of seven to start with. Work with whatever feels most comfortable for you. Perhaps you'll start off counting to four and once that feels good extend it to five. The main point is you start to feel comfortable slowing your breathing down and taking control of the flow. This will help you immeasurably during labour and birth.

When to do it

My suggestion is to practise this type of breathing for five full minutes every morning. If that means setting your alarm five minutes earlier – do it. It's such a great way to start your day and will leave you feeling great as well as preparing you for your labour day, when you'll be using it during each surge you experience.

Birth breathing

Use this technique when you're experiencing a wave or surge when fully dilated.

How to do it

The best way to aid the natural expulsive reflex is to work with the breath in a similar way to when you're wave breathing. The main difference is that you place all of the emphasis on the exhalation. The out-breath needs to be very long and very deep. It can be useful to use a visualization to accompany the out-breath, anything that reminds you of the importance of staying open, relaxed and moving downwards.

Some women use the words 'open, relaxed or release', others will think about there being no resistance, or imagine a flower opening, or will picture something significant to them that helps keep the idea of openness in their mind.

It can be really helpful to work with noise when you're getting to this stage. Although some will feel equally comfortable working with the breath alone, others will want to hum, shout, groan or even moo. If it hasn't already, it can get incredibly primal at this stage. This is nothing for either you or your birth partner to fear. No resistance is the main aim of the game. If you want to howl, just howl! Whatever you instinctively want to do is all good – seriously. The only thing to be mindful of is to use the noise and the energy to send your power back down to your baby and your uterus so they can finish the job.

When to do it

The best place to practise this technique is when you're having a poo. If you're at home, hum when you're on the loo so you start to feel more comfortable and familiar with directing your sound and energy down in that way.

This is great if you're suffering with constipation too. It won't shift everything immediately but by applying patience, the humming and the breathing will see your natural expulsive reflex start to get things moving much more quickly and comfortably.

As mentioned above, use this technique when you're experiencing a wave or surge when you're fully dilated.

Index

About the Authors

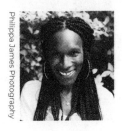

Suzy Ashworth used hypnobirthing to bring her first child, Caesar, into the world. Following a second home water birth with her daughter, Coco, and after speaking to a plethora of women who shared their negative experiences of birth, Suzy developed The Calm Birth Method to help more women understand how they could empower themselves during pregnancy and birth to create more positive birth experiences.

Suzy believes that a woman's birth experience has the power to influence the way she feels about herself, her child and even who she is as an individual. Her Calm Birth Method aims to help women approach birth feeling confident, empowered and knowledgeable, and provides all the tools needed to ensure that a woman's birth experience is both calm and positive. As Suzy says, every mother is a birthing goddess and no one can fail at birth, regardless of the way her baby decides to enter the world.

Suzy holds diplomas in hypnotherapy and psychotherapy. She is a wife, sister, author, speaker, business mentor and mother of three beautiful children.

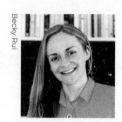

Becky Rui

Liz Stanford used hypnobirthing to birth her two eldest children and, after having two very different experiences (one with intervention and one without), truly felt the power of hypnobirthing. It was this (and the persuasive skills of her husband!) that made her decide to train to teach hypnobirthing in 2011. When Liz came across The Calm Birth School in 2015, after the transformative birth of her third child, she immediately felt connected and aligned to Suzy's message. In 2018 Liz became the proud owner of The Calm Birth School!

Liz believes that hypnobirthing isn't a type of birth but rather a mindset, an approach and a set of tools and techniques that can be applied to any birth experience to help create as positive an experience as possible. She believes that when women and birthing people approach birth with a sense of empowerment, confidence and knowledge they can influence how they will feel about their birth, enabling them to start parenthood in the best possible way.

Liz holds a certification in hypnotherapy, she is a Mindset Coach, an NLP Coach and Practitioner and believes in lifelong learning! She is a wife, mother, daughter, sister, business coach and mentor.

www.thecalmbirthschool.com

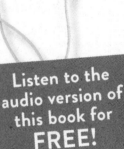
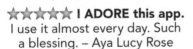

CONNECT WITH
HAY HOUSE
ONLINE

🌐 hayhouse.co.uk   **f** @hayhouse

📷 @hayhouseuk   🐦 @hayhouseuk

▶ @hayhouseuk   ♪ @hayhouseuk

Find out all about our latest books & card decks • Be the first to know about exclusive discounts • Interact with our authors in live broadcasts • Celebrate the cycle of the seasons with us • Watch free videos from your favourite authors • Connect with like-minded souls

'The gateways to wisdom and knowledge are always open.'

Louise Hay